To Kip Smith—
Thank you for the opportunity at the
University of Pittsburgh in 1977 and
for your enduring friendship and support.

Athletic
Taping and Bracing

SECOND EDITION

David H. Perrin, PhD, ATC

University of North Carolina at Greensboro

Human Kinetics

Library of Congress Cataloging-in-Publication Data

Perrin, David H., 1954-
Athletic taping and bracing / David H. Perrin—2nd ed.
p. cm.
Previously published in 1995.
Includes bibliographical references.
ISBN 0-7360-4811-1 (soft cover)
1. Sports injuries--Treatment. 2. Bandages and bandaging. I. Title.
RD97.P47 2005
617.1'027--dc22

2004023781

ISBN-10: 0-7360-4811-1
ISBN-13: 978-0-7360-4811-8

Acquisitions Editor: Loarn D. Robertson, PhD; **Developmental Editor:** Elaine H. Mustain; **Assistant Editor:** Sandra Merz Bott; **Copyeditor:** Bob Replinger; **Proofreader:** Julie Marx Goodreau; **Permission Manager:** Dalene Reeder; **Graphic Designer:** Fred Starbird; **Graphic Artist:** Angela K. Snyder; **Photo Manager:** Kelly J. Huff; **Cover Designer:** Keith Blomberg; **Photographer (cover):** Kelly J. Huff; **Photographer (interior):** Kelly J. Huff; **Art Manager:** Kelly Hendren; **Illustrator:** Primal Pictures, Ltd.; **Printer:** Creative Printing USA

We thank the School of Health and Human Performance at the University of North Carolina at Greensboro for assistance in providing the location for the photo shoot for this book.

We thank Johnson & Johnson for generously supplying tapes used in the photographing of the taping and bracing patterns.

Printed in China.   15   14   13   12   11   10   9

Human Kinetics
Web site: www.HumanKinetics.com

United States: Human Kinetics, P.O. Box 5076, Champaign, IL 61825-5076
800-747-4457
email: humank@hkusa.com

Canada: Human Kinetics, 475 Devonshire Road Unit 100, Windsor, ON N8Y 2L5
800-465-7301 (in Canada only)
email: info@hkcanada.com

Europe: Human Kinetics, 107 Bradford Road, Stanningley, Leeds LS28 6 AT, United Kingdom
+44 (0) 113 255 5665
email: hk@hkeurope.com

Australia: Human Kinetics, 57A Price Avenue, Lower Mitcham, South Australia 5062
08 8372 0999
e-mail: info@hkaustralia.com

New Zealand: Human Kinetics, P.O. Box 80, Torrens Park, South Australia 5062
0800 222 062
e-mail: info@hknewzealand.com

Contents

Preface

Mastering the art and science of athletic taping and bracing requires students of athletic training to develop the psychomotor skills associated with the craft and learn the scientific principles that guide its application. Educators seeking to convey this dual emphasis face the daunting task of teaching students the anatomical architecture of the major joints and muscle groups as well as specific taping and bracing techniques associated with particular injuries.

I wrote *Athletic Taping and Bracing, Second Edition,* as both a guide for instructors and an aid to students. The book includes concise descriptions of anatomy and detailed anatomical illustrations (of the quality usually found in advanced anatomy texts) integrated with discussions of injury mechanisms and nearly 400 photographs depicting the taping and bracing techniques for each major joint and body region. I believe that this approach will not only encourage skill development but also help ensure familiarity with the underlying anatomical landscapes.

Because exercise plays an equally important role in an athlete's safe return to competition, I also include a presentation of the basic stretching and strengthening exercises associated with specific injuries. Although these exercises should not replace other therapeutic methods, they can help the rehabilitated athlete maintain strength and flexibility. The methods I present apply to the athlete who has completed a rehabilitation program and met the criteria for returning to competition. My approach to this material emphasizes that athletic taping and bracing and the associated exercises serve as an adjunct, rather than a panacea, to the athlete's total rehabilitation. By using this multifaceted treatment approach we can minimize an athlete's chance of reinjury. Be advised, however, that rehabilitation and therapeutic exercise are disciplines distinct from the treatments that I discuss in this book.

In chapter 1 I establish athletic taping and bracing (hereafter referred to generally as athletic taping) within the context of the multifaceted practice of athletic training. The chapter stresses the importance of learning anatomy as the foundation to athletic taping and understanding the effect of taping on athletic performance. Students will also learn the necessity of following the rules of the governing sport organizations for the application of tape and braces.

In chapters 2 through 7 I address and illustrate anatomy, injury mechanisms, taping and bracing techniques, and associated stretching and strengthening exercises for each region of the body. Chapter 2 focuses on the foot-ankle-leg complex and, besides presenting several techniques for taping, describes how orthotics can accelerate an injured athlete's return to competition. Chapter 3 overviews the knee and describes the instabilities associated with ligament injury, as well as the role of preventive, rehabilitative, and functional bracing in injury management. Chapter 4 concerns the treatment of hip and thigh injuries, and chapter 5 moves on to the anatomy and injury mechanisms for the shoulder and arm. Chapter 6 presents the techniques available to the clinician when treating the elbow and forearm. Chapter 7 serves a similar purpose for wrist and hand injuries while also presenting the method for splinting tendon ruptures in the fingers.

In this four-color second edition you will find state-of-the-art illustrations of anatomy and injury mechanisms, produced by Primal Pictures, Ltd. The quality of the photography is unsurpassed, and the edges of the tape have been darkened for easier visualization of the taping patterns. Additions in this edition include the technique for making a protective pad from orthoplast, McConnel taping for acromioclavicular joint injury, and several variations to the taping procedures illustrated in the book. Key palpation landmarks have also been identified and illustrated.

Good luck as you embark on your journey into this exciting area of athletic training. The clinician skilled in the art and science of athletic taping quickly earns an athlete's confidence. But becoming proficient at these skills is a challenge, and you should realize that achieving a high level of proficiency comes only after many hours—even years—of practice. I urge you always to visualize the underlying anatomy that you need to support and the mechanism of injury that you seek to prevent. You may feel frustration as you attempt to master these skills. But with concentration and practice, you can become highly adept at athletic taping and bracing.

Acknowledgments

I am indebted to many people for the role they played in the publication of *Athletic Taping and Bracing, Second Edition*. At Human Kinetics, the support of senior acquisitions editor Loarn Robertson; the expertise of developmental editor Elaine Mustain and assistant editor Sandra Merz Bott; and the talent of photographer Kelly Huff, book designer Fred Starbird, and graphic artist Angela K. Snyder enabled the production of a much improved product. At Primal Pictures, Ltd., Canter Martin facilitated the use of Primal imagery for the book, and project manager–editor Jose Barrientos produced the state-of-the art images. At Johnson and Johnson, Jack Weakley provided the supplies used to illustrate the taping and wrapping procedures throughout the book.

Kip Smith served as a consultant for the photoshoot session and helped to illustrate several of the procedures in the book. John Cottone provided excellent suggestions for additional content, and Mary Allen Watson and Tony Kulas helped with the new key palpation landmarks.

Jatin Ambegaonkar, Kimberly Herndon, Tony Kulas, and Yohei Shimokochi enthusiastically served as models for the photo shoot. James Shipp provided access to the University of North Carolina at Greensboro athletic training facility and selected materials and supplies.

CHAPTER 1

Introduction to Taping and Bracing

The National Athletic Trainers' Association Education Council has identified 12 athletic training educational competencies for the health care of the physically active. To become a competent athletic trainer, the student should perfect the cognitive, psychomotor, and affective competencies integral to each domain. These three abilities—which concern the development of knowledge, physical skill, and attitudes toward the athlete and the sport or physical activity in which he or she is engaged—are also necessary for the application of tape and braces. For that reason, I have structured the information in this text using the 12 domains.

Athletic Training Educational Competencies for the Health Care of the Physically Active

1. Risk management and injury prevention
2. Assessment and evaluation
3. Acute care
4. General medical conditions and disabilities
5. Pathology of injury and illness
6. Pharmacological aspects of injury and illness
7. Nutritional aspects of injury and illness
8. Therapeutic exercise
9. Therapeutic modalities
10. Health care administration
11. Professional development and responsibilities
12. Psychosocial intervention and referral

Adapted, by permission, from National Athletic Trainers' Association, 2005, *The 12 Educational Competencies* (Online). Available at www.nataec.org/html/content_areas.html.

ANATOMY AS THE FOUNDATION TO TAPING AND BRACING

A sound understanding of **human anatomy** is necessary for mastering the art and science of taping and bracing. You must understand the anatomical structures that you are attempting to support with the application of tape or a brace. Anyone can learn the psychomotor skills required to tape (the art), but you must also understand the link between the anatomical structure, the mechanism of injury, and the purpose for which tape is applied, such as immobilization, restriction of motion, or support of a ligament or muscle (the science). This book illustrates the most pertinent anatomical structures and mechanisms of injury for each of the body parts that you will learn to support with tape or a brace. You should also be able to identify and palpate these anatomical structures through your understanding of **surface anatomy.** You will find a list of the key palpation landmarks in each chapter of the book.

You will also need to learn and adopt the use of anatomical terminology in describing the position, planes, direction, and movement of the body. The **anatomical position** is the reference

human anatomy—Study of structures and the relationships among structures of the body.

surface anatomy—Study of the form and surface of the body.

anatomical position—Erect position with the arms at the sides and palms of the hands facing forward.

point for use of this terminology. The median plane bisects the body into right and left halves, and any plane parallel to the median plane is the sagittal plane. The coronal plane bisects the body into anterior (toward the front) and posterior (toward the back) portions. The transverse (axial) plane divides the body into superior (upper) and inferior (lower) parts.

In describing the limbs, proximal (closer to) and distal (farther from) identify structures nearer to or farther from the attachment of the limb to the torso. The position of the paired bones of the extremities is often used to describe anatomical location. For example, the thumb is on the radial side of the forearm, and the great toe is on the tibial side of the lower extremity. Palmer and plantar are used to describe the anterior surfaces of the hand and foot, respectively, and dorsal describes the other side in both the hand and foot.

Specific terms also describe movements of the body. Flexion means bending in a direction that usually reduces the angle of a joint, and extension is the opposite movement. Abduction means movement away from the midline, and adduction is the opposite motion. Rotation is movement of a bone around its long axis, and it occurs in the medial (inward) or lateral (outward) direction. Joint-specific terms describe movements at the forearm and foot. Supination and pronation describe movement of the forearm to position the palm up and down, respectively (with the elbow at 90° flexion). Inversion and eversion move the sole of the foot inward or outward, respectively. Circumduction is a combination of movements at joints that permits flexion, abduction, extension, and adduction.

Anatomical Position

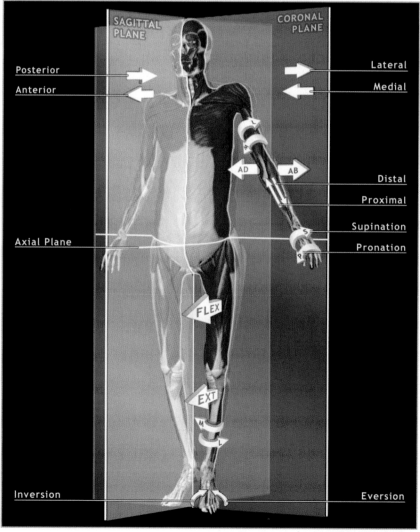

Image courtesy of Primal Pictures.

The taping, wrapping, and bracing techniques that you will learn in this book are designed to support and protect injuries to the bones, ligaments, tendons, muscles, nerves, and joints of the body. Some of the more common injuries for which you will apply tape and wraps are illustrated throughout the text.

Knee Joint

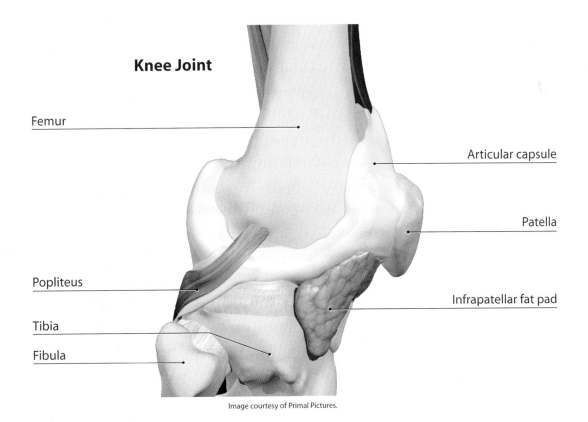

Femur

Articular capsule

Patella

Popliteus

Infrapatellar fat pad

Tibia

Fibula

Image courtesy of Primal Pictures.

Shoulder Complex

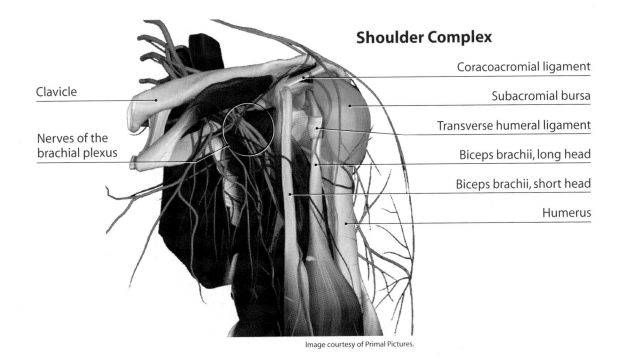

Coracoacromial ligament

Subacromial bursa

Clavicle

Transverse humeral ligament

Nerves of the
brachial plexus

Biceps brachii, long head

Biceps brachii, short head

Humerus

Image courtesy of Primal Pictures.

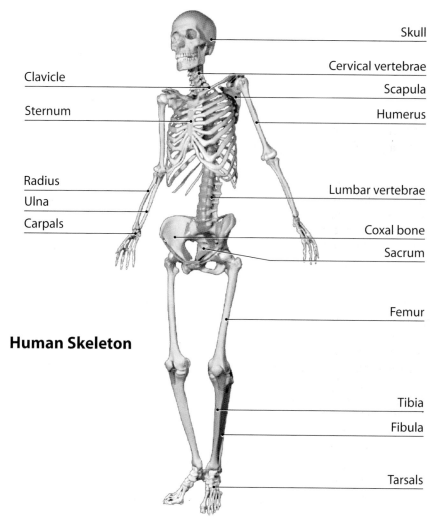

Human Skeleton

Skull
Cervical vertebrae
Scapula
Humerus
Clavicle
Sternum
Lumbar vertebrae
Radius
Ulna
Carpals
Coxal bone
Sacrum
Femur
Tibia
Fibula
Tarsals

Image courtesy of Primal Pictures.

ROLE OF TAPING AND BRACING

Although the National Athletic Trainers' Association's structure for the domains of athletic training lists taping as only one of several abilities necessary for athletic trainers to function effectively, it is one of the most important, and most visible, skills. You can quickly earn an athlete's confidence through proficient application of athletic tape. Learning to master this task, however, will be both rewarding and frustrating. As with any psychomotor skill, taping requires a great deal of practice before one achieves excellence.

Athletic taping and bracing can prevent injury or facilitate an injured athletes' return to competition. In general, the tape should limit abnormal or excessive movement of a **sprained** joint while also providing support to the muscle that the sprain has compromised. Many clinicians attribute the value of taping to the enhanced proprioceptive feedback that the tape provides the athlete during performance. For example, athletes who have injured the anterior cruciate ligament and suffer from rotary instability in the knee may receive sensory cues from the brace before it limits rotary movement. This early **proprioceptive** feedback may enable the athlete subconsciously to contract the muscles that control rotary instability. Similarly, athletes involved in volleyball and basketball may receive sensory cues from a taped ankle that experiences inversion while airborne.

sprain—An overstretching (first degree), partial tearing (second degree), or complete rupture (third degree) of a ligament.

proprioception—Awareness of the position of a body part in space.

Athletic Training Educational Competencies Pertinent to Athletic Taping and Bracing

Risk Management and Injury Prevention

▶ *Cognitive Domain:* Describes the principles and concepts relating to prophylactic taping, wrapping, and bracing and protective pad fabrication.

▶ *Psychomotor Domain:* Selects, fabricates, and applies appropriate preventive taping and wrappings, splints, braces, and other special protective devices that are consistent with sound anatomical and biomechanical principles.

▶ *Affective Domain:* Understands the values and benefits of correctly selecting and using prophylactic taping and wrapping or prophylactic padding.

Therapeutic Exercise

▶ *Cognitive Domain:* Compares the effectiveness of taping, wrapping, bracing, and other supportive and protective methods for facilitation of safe progression to advanced therapeutic exercises and functional activities.

Tape, in this instance, can be more effective in providing proprioceptive feedback than in actually limiting excessive inversion.

Regardless of how tape and braces work, they should not substitute for exercise. Routine taping of the ankle in the absence of preactivity exercise provides the athlete with substandard health care. For this reason, taping should work in conjunction with stretching and strengthening techniques. As a matter of policy, you should tape or brace only those athletes willing to comply with your requests to attain and maintain optimal joint range of motion and muscle strength.

Apparatus of Taping and Bracing

A variety of tools are needed to cover the different taping and bracing needs of injured athletes. These include elastic (figure 1.1) or nonelastic (figure 1.2) athletic tape, cloth, wraps, and braces. Manufacturers produce and market athletic tape in many sizes and textures.

Purposes of Taping and Bracing

▶ Support the ligaments and capsule of unstable joints by limiting excessive or abnormal anatomical movement.

▶ Enhance proprioceptive feedback from the limb or joint.

▶ Support injuries to the muscle-tendon units by compressing and limiting movement.

▶ Secure protective pads, dressings, and splints.

Nonelastic Tape and Cloth

Use nonelastic tape to provide optimal joint support and to restrict abnormal or excessive joint motion. For example, nonelastic white tape applied directly to the ankle can prevent excessive inversion.

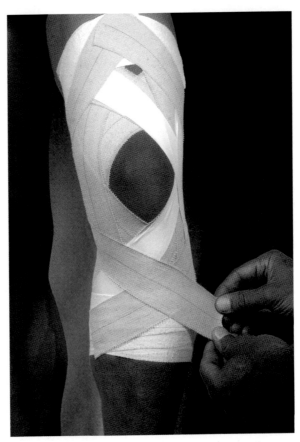

Figure 1.1 Application of elastic tape to support the knee.

Nonelastic white tape is normally porous and is available in 15-yard (13.7-meter) rolls with widths of 1, 1.5, or 2 inches (2.5, 3.8, or 5.1 centimeters). The size of the athlete, the anatomical site, and the preference of the athletic trainer will dictate which width to use.

Although nonelastic tape provides the best support, it has the disadvantage of being the most difficult to use. When applying nonelastic white tape you will find that the contours of the body can easily cause the tape to wrinkle. You will need a great deal of practice to master the smooth and efficient application of nonelastic tape.

Nonelastic cloth wraps can provide support independently or in combination with white tape (figure 1.3). Cloth wraps, although not as convenient as tape, provide acceptable support at considerable cost savings; consider them if your budgetary resources are limited.

Elastic Tape and Wraps

Apply elastic tape or wraps to support body parts that, unlike most joints, require great freedom of movement. For example, when it is necessary to support the hamstring muscle group by encircling the thigh, use elastic tape to permit normal muscle contraction without restricting blood flow. Elastic tape and wraps will also secure protective pads to the body (figure 1.4). An athlete with thigh, hip,

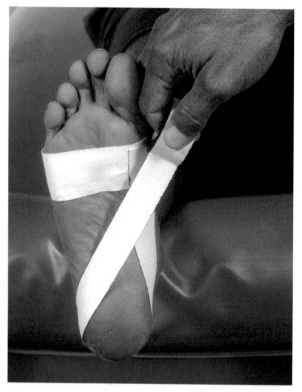

Figure 1.2 Application of nonelastic tape to support the arch.

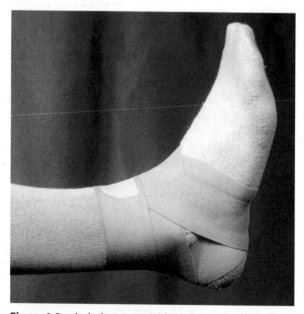

Figure 1.3 A cloth wrap provides inexpensive ankle support. The cloth wrap is also an excellent way to practice the figure-eight and heel-lock techniques presented in chapter 2.

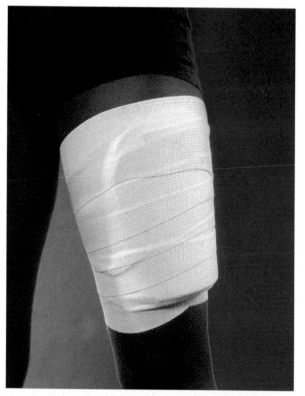

Figure 1.4 An elastic wrap to secure a protective pad to the anterior thigh. The metal clips used to fasten an elastic wrap should be covered with tape or removed for participation.

or shoulder **contusions** often requires this extra protection; I will discuss the technique further in chapters 4 and 5.

Elastic wraps prove especially useful when applying compression to an area that has suffered an **acute injury.** Compression, frequently combined with ice, helps control the swelling that accompanies soft-tissue injuries (figure 1.5).

> **contusion**—A bruise.
>
> **acute injury**—A recent, traumatic injury.

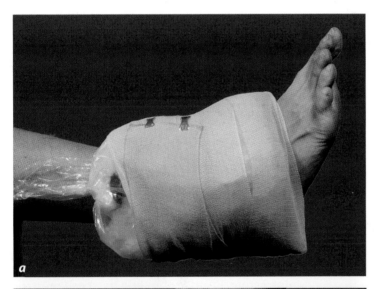

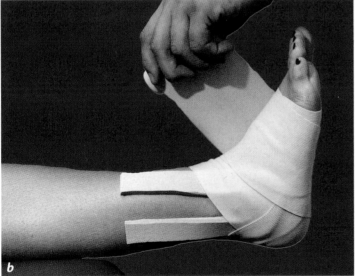

Figure 1.5 *(a)* Elastic wrap to secure an ice bag to the ankle. Apply the ice directly to the skin for no longer than 20 minutes per hour. *(b)* The elastic wrap can also be used in combination with a horseshoe pad to apply compression to an acutely sprained ankle.

When treating athletes with this technique, you should always advise them about the potential risks of applying elastic wraps to acute injuries that will, inevitably, swell. In particular, you should warn the athletes to watch for signs of restricted circulation by monitoring the color of fingernail or toenail beds. A dark blue appearance in a nail bed indicates impaired circulation. If the elastic wrap is necessary, be certain to remind the athlete to elevate the injured joint and apply the wrap loosely if used at night.

Elastic tape, like nonelastic tape, comes in textures and widths for every body part. Elastic tape can be 1, 2, 3, or 4 inches (2.5, 5.1, 7.6, or 10.2 centimeters) wide. Elastic wraps may have widths of 2, 3, 4, or 6 inches (5.1, 7.6, 10.2. or 15.2 centimeters); they are also available in double lengths to accommodate large body areas, such as the hip and trunk. Elastic wrap quality varies. Because you reuse elastic wraps, unlike tape, you could save money by buying the better, often more expensive, product. The cheaper, low-quality wraps do not work well for continued reapplication.

Protective Devices in Combination With Tape and Wraps

Protective splints and pads are frequently used to limit motion, protect a body part, or dissipate forces away from the injured area. Athletic tape and wraps can often be used to hold the protective splints and pads in place. The protective materials include foam, felt, thermoplastics, thermofoams, and other materials such as fiberglass, silicone rubber, and neoprene. The book will provide selected examples of these protective materials and the use of tape and wraps to hold them in place.

Athletic Braces

Braces prevent injury to healthy joints and support unstable joints. A variety of braces is available in the athletic marketplace. In fact, you can find a brace for every joint of the body, although, for athletic purposes, you will most commonly need to apply braces for the ankle, knee, shoulder, elbow, and wrist. I will not supply a comprehensive review of braces; I will focus, instead, on those used to treat common ligament injuries in the ankle and knee, and overuse injuries in the elbow and wrist. In addition, I provide illustrations for ankle, knee, wrist, elbow, and shoulder braces in their respective chapters.

Braces can supplement or replace athletic tape. Some braces, such as those for the ankle, can save money because, unlike athletic tape, they are reusable. Braces, however, can be expensive. Functional knee braces, for example, cost from $500 to $700.

KNOWING THE SPORT, ATHLETE, AND INJURY

To become an effective athletic trainer you must learn both anatomy and the **mechanisms of injury** and master the psychomotor tasks for appropriate athletic taping. In addition, you should understand the rules of the sport regarding taping and bracing and the needs of your individual athletes.

Regulation of Taping and Bracing in Sport

Most governing athletic associations regulate the degree of restriction you can provide through taping and bracing as well as the materials that you use to protect an injured part. They enforce these mandates because the application of tape can give the wearer an unfair advantage during competition, especially in sports such as wrestling. Protective devices and braces can also injure other participants. Most associations prohibit hard and inflexible materials unless you cover them with a soft, pliable padding.

Sport associations also regulate the management of athletic injuries during organized competition. Wrestling, for example, permits only a short time to treat an injured athlete. Many other sports require you to remove the athlete from competition, regardless of the severity of the injury. You must also follow universal precautions if the athlete is bleeding, so you should become very familiar with these procedures. These and other rules affect how you evaluate an injured athlete and apply a brace or tape. I advise you to consult the guidelines of your appropriate governing organization, such as the National Collegiate Athletic Association or a state or regional high school athletic association.

Knowing the Athlete

Some athletes cannot perform with even a small degree of restricted movement, whereas others do quite well with a great deal of limitation. A significant amount of restriction on the hands and fingers of a football offensive or defensive lineman may not inhibit the athlete's performance. In contrast, the same, or lesser, degree of restriction would dramatically compromise the dexterity of a quarterback or receiver. Taping a shot-putter's ankle requires you to use a technique different from the one you apply when supporting the ankle of a sprinter. These examples show that to master the art and science of taping, you must understand the different needs of your athletes.

Examining and Treating the Injury

You must have a thorough mastery of injury assessment and rehabilitation to tape and brace effectively, including knowing when it is safe to return an athlete to practice and competition.

Injury Examination

Under no circumstance should you tape or brace an athlete's injury without first knowing the injury mechanism and its underlying anatomical structure. By understanding the mechanism of injury you will be able to apply tape in a manner that will help prevent further damage. To determine the injury mechanism and know whether the injury is acute or **chronic,** you must obtain an athlete's history. Be systematic in your evaluation by using the injury assessment protocol on page 9. For more information on injury assessment consult the reading list at the end of the book, which includes an excellent text that addresses how to evaluate musculoskeletal injury.

Role of Exercise

As an athletic trainer, you must do more than tape or brace an injured athlete; you have a responsibility to provide the athlete with appropriate stretching and strengthening exercises. Preventing injury or eliminating its recurrence will be possible only when the athlete has achieved normal strength, flexibility, and range of motion! I discuss in this book exercises that require minimal equipment. Have the rehabilitated athlete who has met the criteria for returning to competition use them to maintain strength and flexibility.

Criteria for Returning to Competition

Although taping procedures facilitate an athlete's return to physical activity, these adjunctive measures do not substitute for the athlete's preinjury functional ability. When athletes suffer an upper- or lower-extremity injury, they should possess strength, flexibility, and range of motion comparable to the uninjured side before continuing with the sport. If the injury involves the lower extremity, test the athlete on functional activities that include running and cutting. For example, an athlete displaying an **antalgic gait**, with or without tape, should not return to competition.

---

mechanism of injury—Describes the specific cause of the injury.

chronic injury—A nontraumatic injury of an ongoing nature.

antalgic gait—A painful or abnormal walking or running pattern.

Injury Assessment Protocol

► Obtain the athlete's history relating to the mechanism of injury.

► Inspect the area for swelling and deformity.

► Palpate the part for abnormalities.

► Assess the active range of motion—the athlete's willingness to move the part.

► Determine the passive range of motion—your ability to move the part while the athlete relaxes.

► Evaluate the resistive range of motion—the athlete's ability to contract the muscles about the part.

► Apply special tests to assess the integrity of the ligaments of the joint.

► Always compare your findings with the uninjured extremity!

PREPARING FOR TAPING

Taping should occur in an environment that maximizes your effectiveness. Because you will

Criteria for Returning an Injured Athlete to Competition

► The injured area has regained normal strength, flexibility, and range of motion when compared with the uninjured side.

► The athlete performs functional tests, such as running, cutting, and other agility exercises, at full speed without limping.

► The athlete's psychological condition demonstrates willingness and enthusiasm to return.

---

devote many hours to this psychomotor task, you will optimize your clinical taping skills by preparing yourself, your facility, and your athletes. Your preparation and the athlete's cooperation are essential.

Taping Environment

Maintain the cleanliness and professional appearance of your taping area. It should have adequate illumination and ventilation. Because heat and humidity make it difficult to apply tape, store your supplies in a cool environment.

Your work will require you to spend many hours performing psychomotor skills. Therefore, construct the taping environment and use a taping table to ensure your comfort. Taping tables differ from treatment tables. In general, treatment tables are 72 inches (183 centimeters) long and 30 inches (76 centimeters) high; taping tables should be approximately 48 inches (122 centimeters) long and 35 inches (89 centimeters) high, depending on the clinician's height.

When traveling with a team, arrange an adequate facility for pregame taping. Taping from a bus seat or hotel bed can turn this pleasurable routine into an arduous and painful process.

Gender Considerations

Athletic training has attained the status of an allied health profession, and athletes should be treated in a coeducational environment. In most practice settings you will care for both male and female athletes. Taping an opposite-gender athlete rarely presents any difficulty, but you should always protect your athletes' privacy. For example, the female athlete should wear a halter top or jog

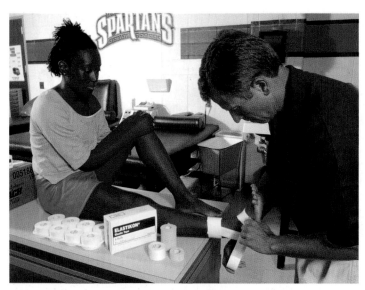

Figure 1.6 Attentive athlete during ankle taping. Note how the athlete sits with the ankle held at 90°.

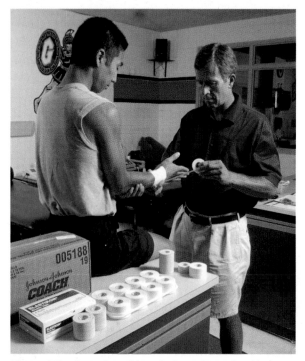

Figure 1.7 Attentive athlete during wrist taping. Note how the athlete stabilizes the forearm while the athletic trainer applies tape to the wrist.

bra during shoulder taping, and you can apply elastic wraps over tights to the hip and groin in both male and female athletes.

Team travel away from home occasionally creates an inconvenience when preparing an area for pregame taping, and the difficulty sometimes increases when caring for opposite-gender athletes. You have the option of waiting for athletes

to be properly clothed before entering the locker room to fulfill your taping responsibilities. Should time become a consideration, have the taping table removed from the locker room to an adjacent area. You can then tape your athletes while the remainder of the team dresses for competition.

Preparation and Cooperation of the Athlete

Athletes should sit or stand and pay attention when you tape the injured area (figures 1.6 and 1.7). An inattentive athlete who is slouching or reclining on the taping table will fail to maintain the injured body part in an appropriate anatomical position. A sagging ankle or limp wrist will quickly cause you frustration and compromise the effectiveness of your procedure.

Before applying tape, make certain that the area is clean and, ideally, free of hair. Keep a barber's clipper handy in your taping area.

You may use an additional adherent when applying tape—many are available commercially—but it is not necessary if the body part is clean, shaved, and dry. When tape contacts bone prominences and muscle tendons, the resulting friction often produces blisters. To maximize the athlete's comfort, apply friction pads with lubricant to these areas before using tape (figure 1.8). Pretaping underwrap may also prevent blistering, but it often causes the tape to slip (figure 1.9). For this reason, I recommend a minimal amount of underwrap, applied in conjunction with tape adherent.

APPLYING AND REMOVING TAPE

Here are several basic skills you must learn when applying and removing tape:

• **Tearing tape:** Although a seemingly simple task, tearing tape will present your first challenge. Developing this skill is often frustrating, particularly when your instructor prohibits you from using your teeth! To tear tape successfully, place your fingers close together at the site of the intended tear, pull the tape apart, and quickly snap your fingers in opposite directions (figure 1.10). If the tape becomes crimped or folded, its tensile strength increases exponentially, and it will be impossible to tear. If this occurs, move to

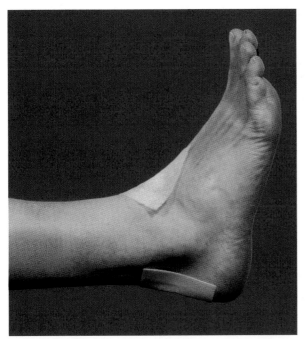

Figure 1.8   Friction pads placed over bony prominences or areas prone to irritation from tape. Place these pads over the tendons in the front and back of the ankle before taping to prevent cuts and abrasions.

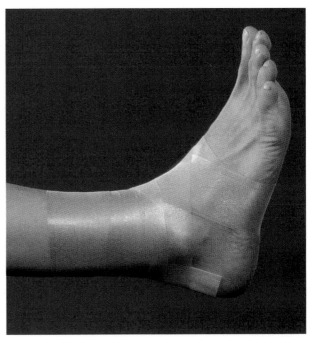

Figure 1.9   Underwrap before tape application. For optimal adherence, apply the tape directly to the skin. For some athletes, however, underwrap can prevent irritation or rashes that may result from the prolonged contact of tape with skin.

a different point along the edge of the tape and try again.

• **Applying tape:** Begin taping by first supplying anchors that will secure the subsequent strips (figure 1.11). As you apply the tape, overlap the previous strip by one-half the width of the tape (figure 1.12). Whenever possible, tape from the **distal** to the **proximal** points of an extremity, using single strips. Avoid continuously unwind-

ing the tape around an extremity because this technique may produce wrinkles and compromise circulation.

distal—A point on an extremity located away from the trunk.

proximal—A point on an extremity located near the trunk.

Figure 1.10   Technique for tearing nonelastic tape. (a) Place the fingers close together and follow with a quick, snapping motion in opposite directions. (b) The tape should tear, but if it becomes folded or crimped, move your fingers away from the folded area and try again. You can tear some elastic tape with the fingers, but you will need to cut other types with scissors.

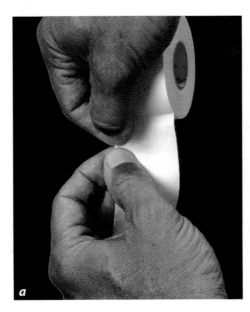

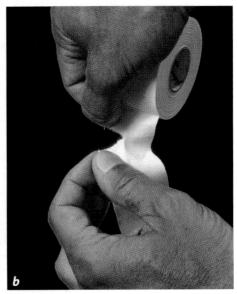

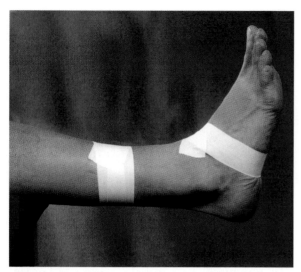

Figure 1.11   Application of anchor strips to start most taping procedures, illustrating anchor strips on the ankle before taping. Note the potential for irritation over the ankle tendons because of the absence of friction pads.

• **Removing Tape:** Athletic trainers should be sure to remove all tape at the conclusion of practices or games. Use surgical scissors or commercially available tape cutters to cut the tape in an area with the least bone prominence and greatest tissue compliance (figure 1.13). Pull back the tape with a slow, gentle motion while the skin is compressed (figure 1.14). Tape-removing agents are available to ease the process. You should monitor the skin for cuts, blisters, or signs of allergic reaction. Properly clean and dress cuts and blisters. If the athlete develops a rash, you will need to find an alternative to treating the injury with tape.

I've included this general competency checklist to help instructors and students alike evaluate the knowledge, skills, and techniques necessary for effective injury assessment and taping.

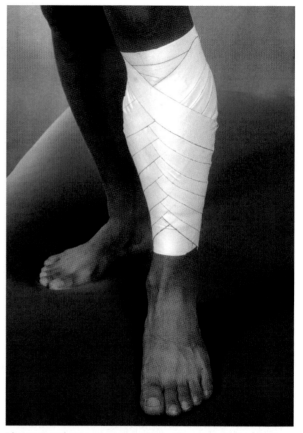

Figure 1.12   Overlapping strips of tape applied to the leg. Note how each strip overlaps the preceding strip by one-half the width of the tape. Tear each strip after application rather than apply the tape in a continuous fashion. Continuously applying nonelastic tape usually produces wrinkles and can constrict blood flow and normal muscle function. Normally, you may apply elastic tape and elastic wraps in a continuous manner.

The principles I have presented in this chapter will prepare you for the specific treatments that I discuss in the remaining chapters. Good luck as you begin your training in these gratifying psychomotor skills!

Taping Competency Checklist

1. Determines mechanism of injury: ☐
2. Ensures a clean, shaved body part: ☐
3. Selects appropriate tape or wrap: ☐
4. Properly positions athlete and body part: ☐
5. Correctly applies appropriate taping procedure: ☐
6. Correctly instructs athlete on tape removal: ☐
7. Ensures the athlete's compliance with appropriate exercise regimen: ☐

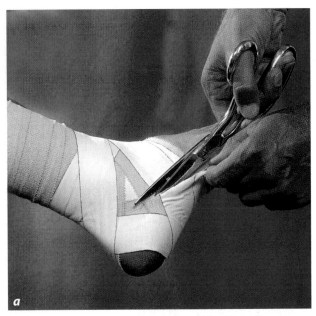

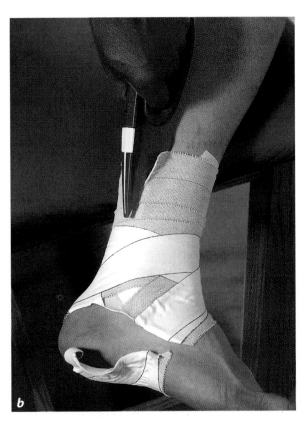

Figure 1.13 *(a)* Use surgical scissors with a blunt tip or a tape cutter to remove tape. *(b)* Cut the tape where it tends to be loose because of the anatomical configuration of the body part.

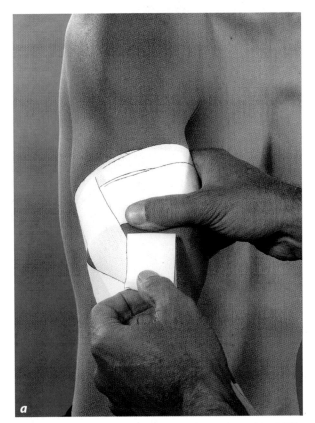

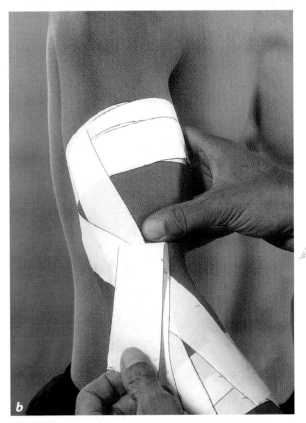

Figure 1.14 Appropriate removal of tape from skin. *(a)* Note how one hand supports the skin while the other *(b)* slowly removes the tape by pulling in a direction exactly opposite the stabilized skin.

CHAPTER 2

The Foot, Ankle, and Leg

The foot contains a complex collection of bones, ligaments, and muscles. The 26 bones of the foot create several important joints. The talus and calcaneus form the subtalar joint, and the joining of the calcaneus with the cuboid and the talus with the navicular creates the midtarsal joint. The base of the five metatarsal bones and the tarsal bones form the tarsometatarsal (TMT) joints, while the heads of the metatarsals and the phalanges form the metatarsophalangeal

Bones of the Foot

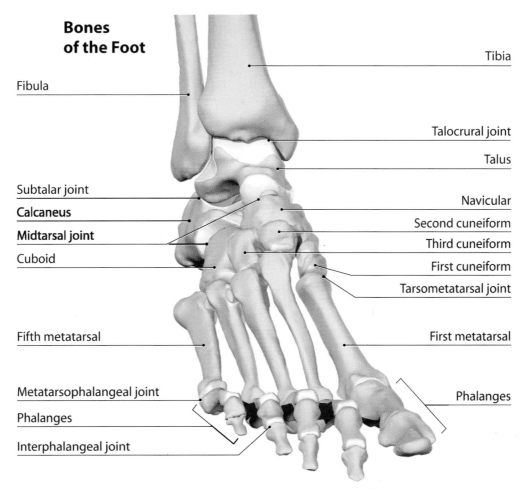

Fibula

Tibia

Talocrural joint

Talus

Subtalar joint

Calcaneus

Navicular

Midtarsal joint

Second cuneiform

Cuboid

Third cuneiform

First cuneiform

Tarsometatarsal joint

Fifth metatarsal

First metatarsal

Metatarsophalangeal joint

Phalanges

Phalanges

Interphalangeal joint

Image courtesy of Primal Pictures.

(MP) joints. Each of the toes contains interphalangeal joints—one interphalangeal joint in the great toe and a proximal (PIP) and distal (DIP) interphalangeal joint in the remaining four toes. A multitude of small ligaments supports the joints in the foot.

The bones of the foot also create two arches. The first, a longitudinal arch, appears along the **medial** border of the foot. Athletes with a pronounced (high) longitudinal arch are **pes cavus,** whereas those with flat feet have a **pes planus** foot. The second arch, formed by the heads of the five metatarsal bones, is the transverse arch.

The foot contains four muscle layers, known collectively as **intrinsic muscles.** The most **superficial** layer, the plantar fascia, maintains the longitudinal arch of the foot. The medial and **lateral** plantar nerves **innervate** the intrinsic muscles. These nerves continue into the toes between the metatarsal heads as **interdigital** nerves and are a common point of irritation in athletes.

medial—Toward the inside.

pes cavus—A foot with a high longitudinal arch.

pes planus—A foot with a flat longitudinal arch.

intrinsic muscle—A muscle that originates and inserts within the foot or hand.

superficial—Toward the surface of the body.

lateral—Toward the outside.

innervation—The process of sending a nerve impulse from the central nervous system to the periphery to induce a muscle to contract.

interdigital—Located between the digits (i.e., the fingers and toes).

The **articulation** of the distal tibia and fibula with the talus, known as the talocrural joint, forms the ankle. The ankle and foot move by using a combination of the talocrural, subtalar, and midtarsal joints. Ankle **dorsiflexion** and **plantar flexion** occur primarily at the talocrural joint; **inversion** and **eversion** take place at the subtalar joint (figure 2.1). Foot **abduction** and **adduction** occur at the midtarsal joint. A combination (while non–weight bearing) of ankle dorsiflexion, eversion, and foot abduction causes **pronation;** plantar flexion, inversion, and adduction result in **supination.**

articulation—The point where two or more adjacent bones create a joint.

dorsiflexion—Movement of the foot toward the upper, or dorsal, surface.

plantar flexion—Movement of the foot toward the bottom, or plantar, surface.

inversion—Inward movement, or turning, of the foot.

eversion—Outward movement, or turning, of the foot.

abduction—Movement away from the midline of the body.

adduction—Movement toward the midline of the body.

pronation—Movement of the forearm to place the palm facedown; or, while non–weight bearing, a combination of dorsiflexion, eversion, and foot abduction.

supination—Movement of the forearm to place the palm faceup; or, while non–weight bearing, a combination of plantar flexion, inversion, and foot adduction.

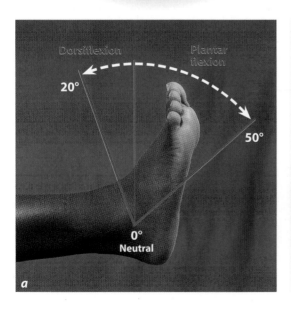

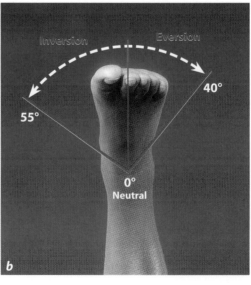

Figure 2.1
(a) Ankle plantar flexion and dorsiflexion ranges of motion; *(b)* ankle inversion and eversion ranges of motion.

Several ligaments reinforce the ankle. On the lateral side, the **anterior** talofibular, calcaneofibular, and posterior talofibular ligaments prevent excessive inversion. The broad and expansive deltoid ligament—a combination of four ligaments—provides stability to the medial aspect of the ankle and checks excessive eversion.

Extrinsic muscles acting on the toes and ankle have their **origin** in the leg. The anterior muscles—the tibialis anterior, extensor hallucis longus, extensor digitorum longus, and peroneus tertius—produce dorsiflexion and toe extension. The lateral muscles, consisting of the peroneus longus and peroneus brevis, cause eversion. The deep posterior-medial muscles, which include the tibialis posterior, flexor hallucis longus, and flexor digitorum longus, produce inversion and toe flexion. Plantar flexion occurs from the gastrocnemius, soleus, and plantaris muscles, also known as true **posterior** muscles. The gastrocnemius and soleus join with the calcaneus to form the Achilles tendon. The gastrocnemius and plantaris begin above the knee, but the soleus originates in the leg. This distinction will be significant during the discussion of stretching exercises for the ankle.

The ankle contains several **retinacula** that hold the tendons of the extrinsic muscles to the leg as they cross the ankle and pass into the foot. The extensor retinacula will be relevant when you use tape to alleviate the discomfort of shin splints.

> **anterior**—The front or top surface of a limb.
>
> **extrinsic muscle**—A muscle that originates in the leg or forearm and inserts into the foot or hand.
>
> **origin**—The point where muscle attaches to bone; usually refers to the proximal attachment of the muscle.
>
> **posterior**—The rear or bottom surface of a limb.
>
> **retinaculum**—A soft-tissue fibrous structure designed to stabilize tendons or bones.

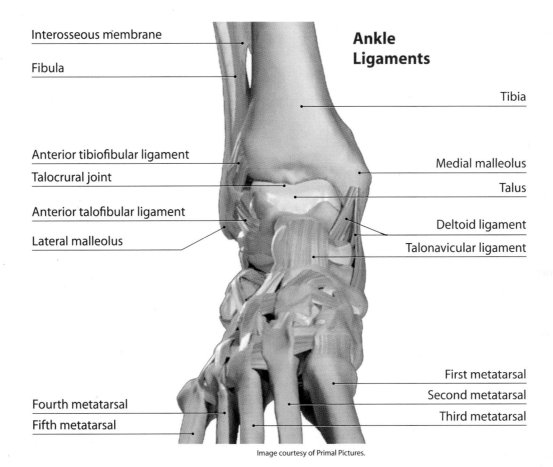

Ankle Ligaments

Interosseous membrane

Fibula

Tibia

Anterior tibiofibular ligament

Talocrural joint

Anterior talofibular ligament

Lateral malleolus

Medial malleolus

Talus

Deltoid ligament

Talonavicular ligament

First metatarsal

Second metatarsal

Third metatarsal

Fourth metatarsal

Fifth metatarsal

Image courtesy of Primal Pictures.

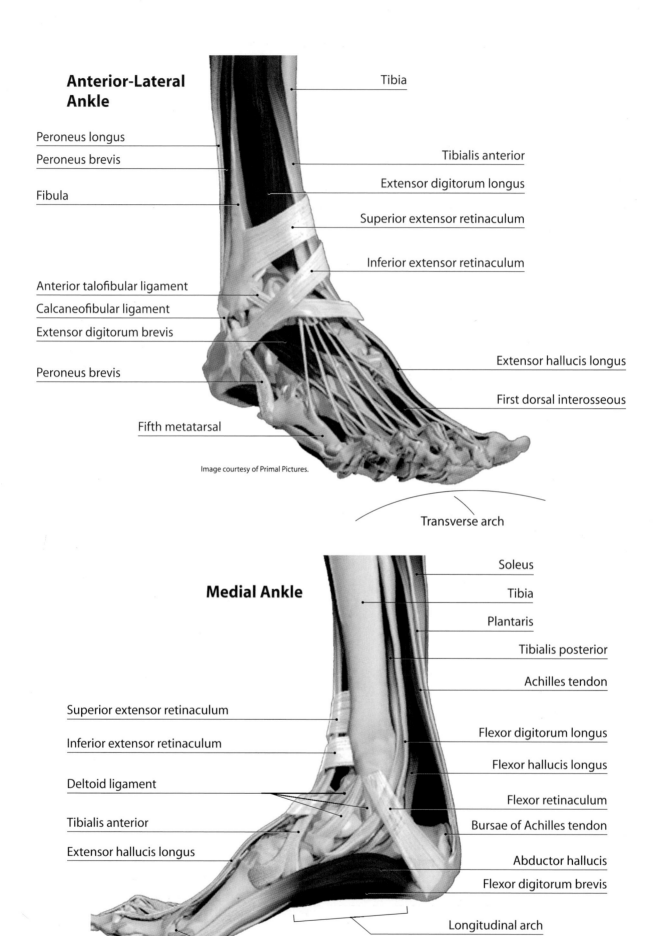

Anterior-Lateral Ankle

Peroneus longus

Peroneus brevis

Fibula

Anterior talofibular ligament

Calcaneofibular ligament

Extensor digitorum brevis

Peroneus brevis

Fifth metatarsal

Tibia

Tibialis anterior

Extensor digitorum longus

Superior extensor retinaculum

Inferior extensor retinaculum

Extensor hallucis longus

First dorsal interosseous

Image courtesy of Primal Pictures.

Transverse arch

Medial Ankle

Superior extensor retinaculum

Inferior extensor retinaculum

Deltoid ligament

Tibialis anterior

Extensor hallucis longus

Soleus

Tibia

Plantaris

Tibialis posterior

Achilles tendon

Flexor digitorum longus

Flexor hallucis longus

Flexor retinaculum

Bursae of Achilles tendon

Abductor hallucis

Flexor digitorum brevis

Longitudinal arch

First metacarpophalangeal joint

Image courtesy of Primal Pictures.

Posterior Muscles

Gastrocnemius

Achilles tendon

Plantaris

Peroneus brevis

Peroneus longus

Flexor hallucis longus

Calcaneus

Image courtesy of Primal Pictures.

Key Palpation Landmarks

Lateral Aspect
▸ Anterior talofibular ligament
▸ Calcaneofibular ligament
▸ Posterior talofibular ligament

Medial Aspect
▸ Deltoid ligament
▸ Longitudinal arch

Anterior Aspect
▸ Anterior tibiofibular ligament

Posterior Aspect
▸ Achilles tendon
▸ Gastrocnemius muscle
▸ Soleus muscle

Plantar Surface
▸ Plantar fascia
▸ Transverse arch
▸ Calcaneus

Dorsal Surface
▸ First metatarso-phalangeal joint

Surface Anatomy

Tibia

Tibialis anterior

Flexor digitorum longus

Medial malleolus

Sustentaculum tali

Abductor hallucis

Tuberosity of navicular

Head of first metatarsal

Extensor hallucis longus

Extensor digitorum longus

Image courtesy of Primal Pictures.

(continued)

(continued)

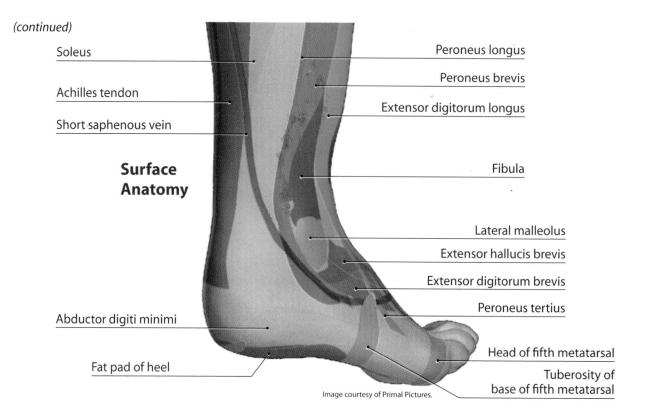

Surface Anatomy

Soleus

Achilles tendon

Short saphenous vein

Abductor digiti minimi

Fat pad of heel

Peroneus longus

Peroneus brevis

Extensor digitorum longus

Fibula

Lateral malleolus

Extensor hallucis brevis

Extensor digitorum brevis

Peroneus tertius

Head of fifth metatarsal

Tuberosity of base of fifth metatarsal

Image courtesy of Primal Pictures.

ANKLE SPRAINS

Physical activity places excessive stress on the foot and ankle and renders this region of the body highly susceptible to injury. Ankle sprains will be the most common injury that you encounter.

Ankle sprains result from excessive inversion or eversion. Inversion sprains are more common because of the bone and ligament configuration of the joint. The four ligaments of the deltoid complex are stronger than the three separate, laterally placed ligaments, and the mortise created by the fibula extends more distally than the tibia. These factors limit eversion and account for the higher incidence of inversion ankle sprains. You can support the sprained ankle by applying tape, braces, or a combination of the two treatments.

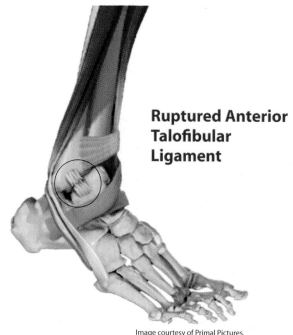

Ruptured Anterior Talofibular Ligament

Image courtesy of Primal Pictures.

Closed Basketweave Taping

Begin the closed basketweave procedure by applying anchor strips and follow with a succession of interlocking vertical and horizontal strips. Complete the taping with one or more heel-lock strips on the medial and lateral aspects of the ankle (figure 2.2). With an inversion sprain, start the vertical strips on the medial side of the leg and pull to the lateral aspect. For an eversion injury, begin the vertical strips on the lateral leg and pull to the medial side. Note that horizontal and vertical strips pertain to the anatomical position of the body (i.e., standing erect).

Be aware that applying an anchor too tight around the foot is the most frequent error with this taping procedure. Because the foot spreads when supporting the weight of the body, a constricting distal anchor can be extremely uncomfortable for an athlete. Apply this anchor as close to the ankle as possible. You can even omit it for athletes requiring greater dexterity.

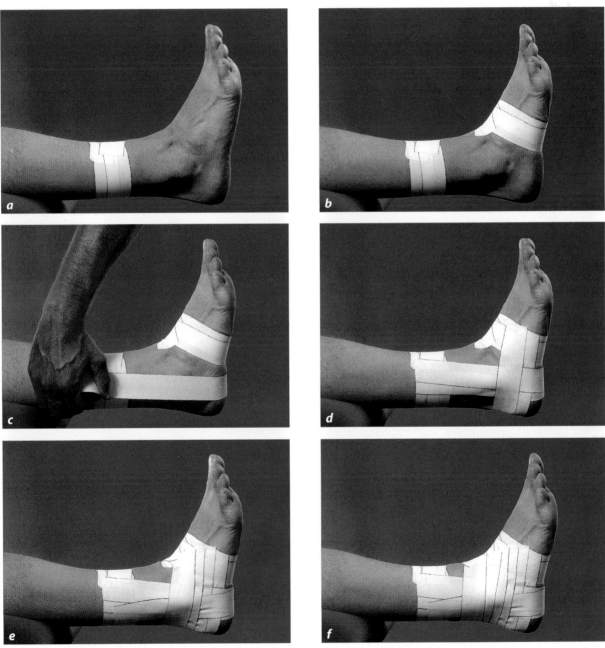

Figure 2.2   Closed basketweave taping procedure for the ankle. The athlete holds the ankle in 90° of dorsiflexion. For ease of illustration, these photos do not show the use of friction pads. Place two anchor strips on *(a)* the distal leg and, possibly, *(b)* around the foot. Because the foot anchors frequently cause constriction and discomfort, consider them optional. To prevent or protect inversion sprains, *(c)* apply a stirrup strip from the medial aspect of the leg and pull under the heel to the lateral aspect of the leg. For eversion sprains, the direction of the stirrup would be the opposite, from lateral leg to medial leg. Place a horizontal horseshoe strip from the medial to lateral aspect of the foot and *(d)* follow by another stirrup in a weaving fashion. *(e-f)* Continue this process until you have applied three stirrups.

(continued)

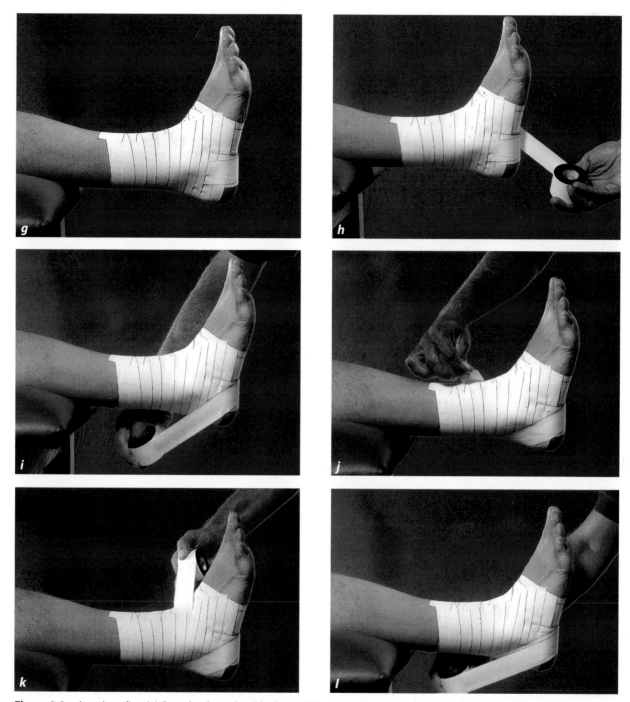

Figure 2.2 *(continued)* *(g)* Completely enclose the leg with horizontal strips. *(h-j)* Apply heel locks to the medial and lateral aspects of the ankle in a single manner (application to the lateral side of the ankle is shown here). Note how to apply the lateral heel lock by pulling in an upward direction. *(k-n)* A more advanced variation would incorporate heel locks in a figure-eight pattern. Note how to apply the lateral heel lock by pulling in an upward direction and the medial heel lock by pulling in a downward direction. *(continued)*

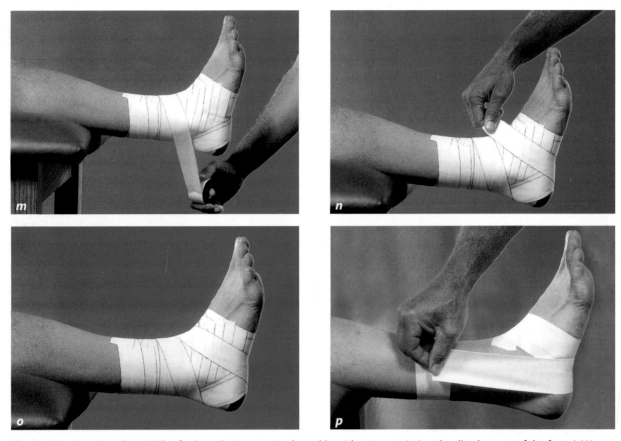

Figure 2.2 *(continued)* *(o)* The final product supports the ankle without constricting the distal aspect of the foot. *(p)* You can provide additional support with the application of a 2- or 3-inch (5.1- or 7.6-centimeter) moleskin stirrup before applying the closed basketweave.

Taping Variations and Alternatives

Purchase large rolls of cloth wrap that can be cut into lengths of 72 inches (about 180 centimeters).

Combining the cloth wrap with a small amount of white tape will provide adequate support (figure 2.3). Cloth wraps do not work as well as nonelastic tape, but they are a reasonable, cost-effective alternative.

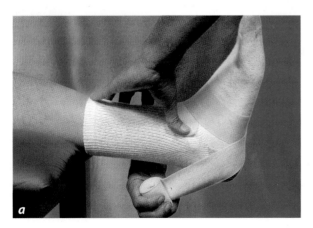
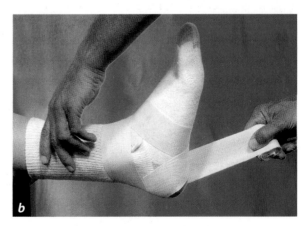

Figure 2.3 Apply a cloth ankle wrap as a less expensive (although less effective) alternative to closed basketweave taping. Apply this procedure over a sock with the ankle positioned in 90° of dorsiflexion. First, *(a-b)* use a figure-eight pattern with heel locks incorporated in an upward direction for the lateral aspect and a downward direction for the medial aspect.

(continued)

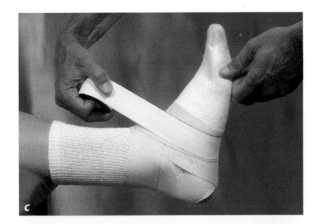

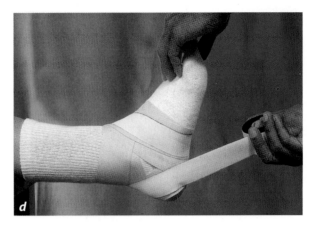

Figure 2.3 *(continued)*
(c-e) Trace with nonelastic tape.

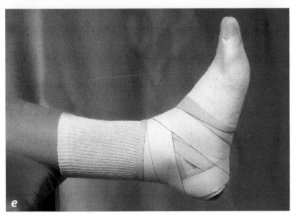

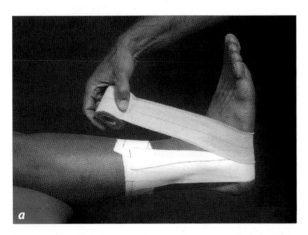

You can also use the closed basketweave procedure with a combination of moleskin (figure 2.2) or nonelastic and elastic tape (figure 2.4). This alternative may be acceptable for athletes who want some protection but do not require the additional support of an all-white taping procedure.

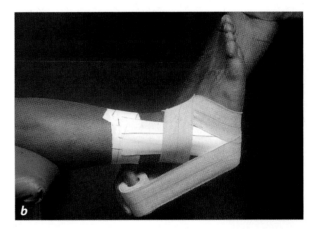

Figure 2.4 Nonelastic and elastic tape combination. For less support, *(a-b)* use stirrups of nonelastic tape and apply both a figure-eight pattern and heel locks with elastic tape.

(continued)

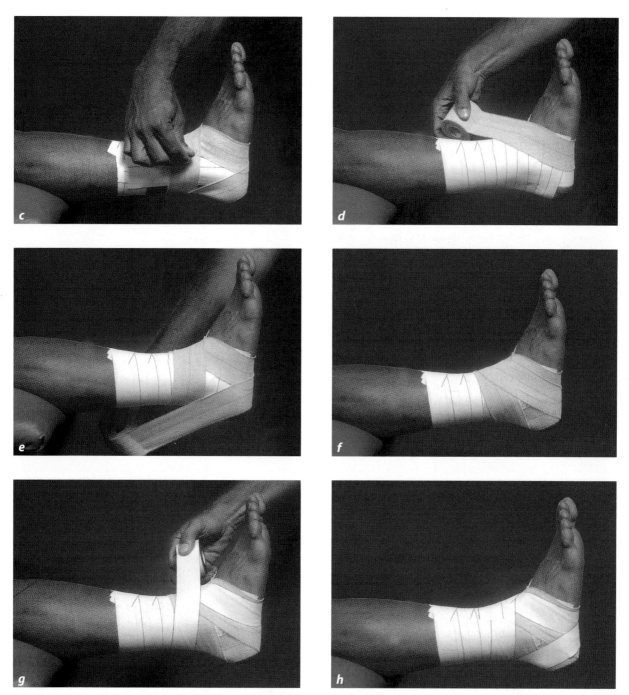

Figure 2.4 *(continued (c)* Use elastic tape to encircle the leg completely to the anchor strips; you then have the option of repeating the figure eight and heel locks with nonelastic tape. *(d-f)* A variation that would provide additional support uses nonelastic tape for all stirrup and horseshoe strips and then includes elastic tape to apply the figure eight and heel locks. *(g-h)* Elastic tape could complete the procedure, or you could repeat the figure eight and heel locks with nonelastic tape.

Open Basketweave Taping

This taping technique supports and compresses the acutely injured ankle. Although similar to the closed basketweave, the open technique leaves the **dorsum** of the foot uncovered (figure 2.5). In some cases, you can cover the taping procedure with an elastic wrap to supply more compression. Instruct the athlete to remove the elastic wrap at night but to leave the taping procedure in place.

> **dorsum**—The top of the foot or the back of the hand.

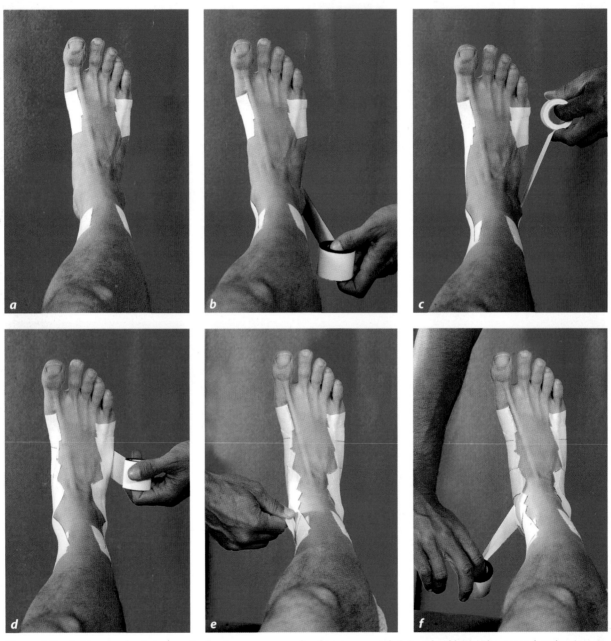

Figure 2.5   Ankle open basketweave taping to compress and support an acutely injured ankle. *(a)* The procedure begins with proximal and distal anchors, but leave them open on the anterior leg and the dorsum of the foot. *(b)* For an inversion sprain, pull the stirrup strips from the medial to lateral aspects of the leg. *(c)* Apply the horseshoe strips in a manner similar to the closed basketweave, giving special attention to leaving the anterior leg and dorsum of the foot open. *(d-e)* Apply stirrups and horseshoe strips to enclose completely the plantar surface of the foot and the posterior aspect of the leg. Use single heel locks for *(f)* the medial and *(g)* lateral ankle.

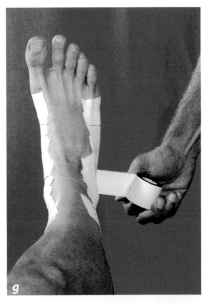

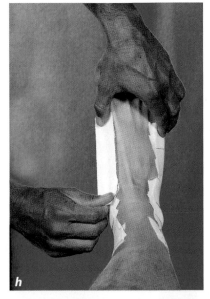

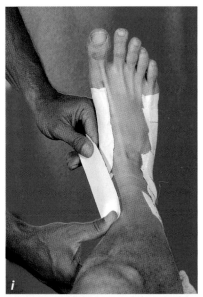

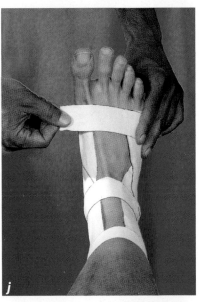

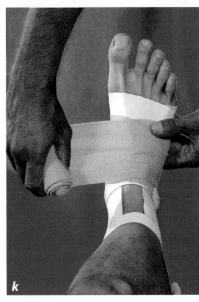

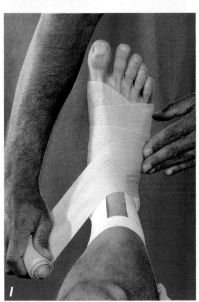

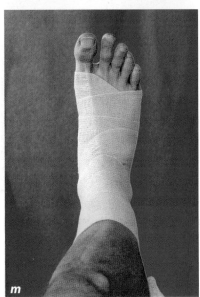

Figure 2.5 *(continued)*
(h-i) Apply anchor strips to the anterior leg and dorsum of the foot. *(j)* Three horizontal strips secure the procedure, although you should instruct the athlete to remove these strips if the ankle begins to ache from significant swelling. *(k-m)* Finally, apply an elastic wrap to secure the open basketweave and to offer additional compression to the acutely injured ankle. Remove the wrap when applying ice and when the athlete sleeps.

Because you apply the open basketweave taping procedure to support an acutely sprained ankle, you also may have to fit and provide the athlete with crutches. The crutches should be fit so that they are 6 inches (15.2 centimeters) lateral and anterior to the feet and permit two to three finger widths of space between the axillae and the axillary pads of the crutches. The elbows should be flexed to about 20 to 30°, and you should instruct the athlete to bear most of the weight with the hands, not in the axillae (figure 2.6).

Ankle Braces

Lace braces have become a popular substitute for ankle tape, especially when a clinician is unavailable (figure 2.7). These commercial supports can also supplement the taping procedure. The brace, normally applied over the sock, often uses lateral stays for reinforcement.

Ankle Exercises

Ankle exercises should restore or maintain normal flexibility, strength, and balance. A loss of normal ankle dorsiflexion often results from ankle sprains. Athletes recovering from these injuries should stretch the ankle muscles and pay special attention to the gastrocnemius and soleus.

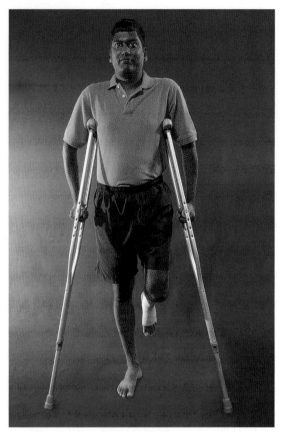

Figure 2.6　An athlete with an antalgic gait should be fitted with crutches. The hands, not the axillae, should bear most of the weight.

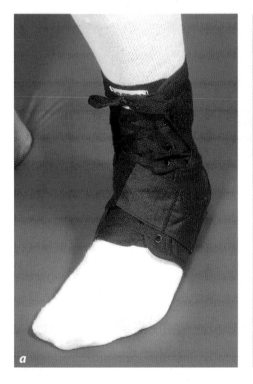

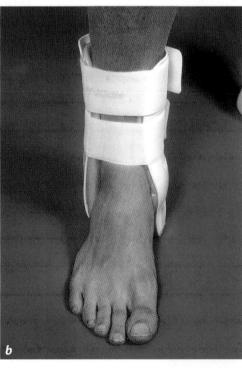

Figure 2.7　*(a-b)* Commercially available ankle braces that are alternatives to taping. The brace permits normal plantar flexion and dorsiflexion while limiting excessive inversion and eversion.

Figure 2.8 illustrates techniques for stretching the gastrocnemius and soleus muscles. Because the gastrocnemius begins on the femur, the athlete first stretches with the knee completely extended. The athlete continues by repeating the exercise with the knee flexed. The flexed knee shortens the gastrocnemius and isolates the soleus muscle, which originates from the tibia and fibula. Using a wedge board will also effectively stretch these muscles. The athlete can manually stretch the remaining ankle muscles. Instruct your athletes to perform **static stretching**—a stretch without movement for 10 to 15 seconds—for these and all exercises that I present in this book.

static stretching—Stretching a muscle in a stationary position.

Strengthening exercises for the major muscle groups acting on the ankle implement elastic bands. The athlete simply performs inversion, eversion, plantar flexion, and dorsiflexion against the resistance of the band (figure 2.9). The methods for strengthening the ankle are similar to stretching exercises. The athlete should execute plantar flexion with the knee both extended and flexed to isolate the gastrocnemius and soleus, respectively. I suggest that the athlete complete three sets of at least 10 repetitions, with resistance adjusted to his or her tolerance, for all the strengthening exercises in this book. The reading list provides references to more sophisticated protocols for progressive resistance exercise.

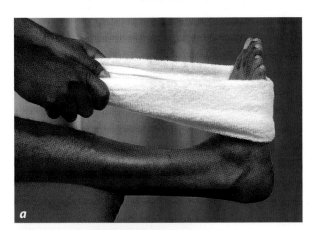

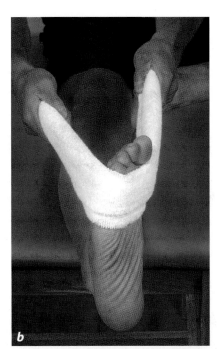

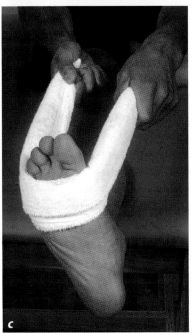

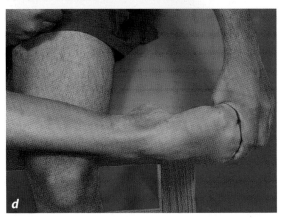

Figure 2.8 *(a)* Stretching the gastrocnemius leg muscle using a towel. The athlete should dorsiflex the ankle with his or her own muscles and use the towel to provide an additional stretch. This stretch should also combine *(b)* ankle inversion and *(c)* eversion; repeat all three stretches with the knee flexed to 90° and with the leg hanging over the end of the table to isolate the soleus muscle. *(d)* Stretch the anterior ankle muscles by having the athlete manually move the ankle into plantar flexion.

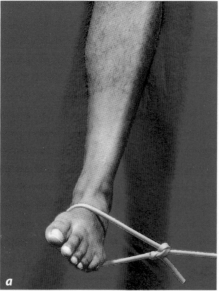
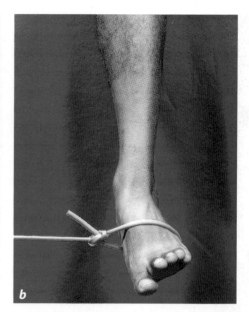

Figure 2.9 Ankle strengthening exercises with elastic material. Move the ankle into (a) inversion, (b) eversion, (c) plantar flexion, and (d) dorsiflexion against the resistance of the material. (e) Repeat plantar flexion with the knee flexed to 90° to isolate the soleus muscle.

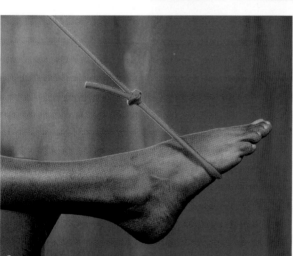
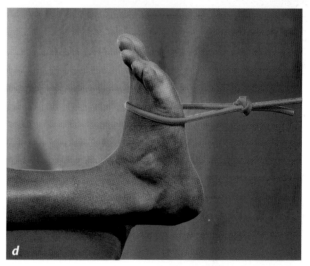

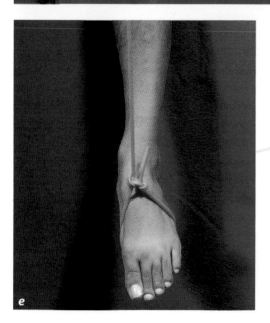

An ankle injury will often compromise an athlete's balance and proprioception. Balance devices are available to address these problems. You can also treat balance and proprioception deficits by having the athlete stand on one leg with the eyes open and then closed (figure 2.10). Increase the difficulty of this exercise by applying light pressure to the shoulders from four random directions when the athlete's eyes are shut.

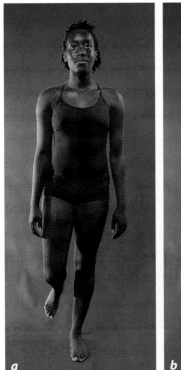
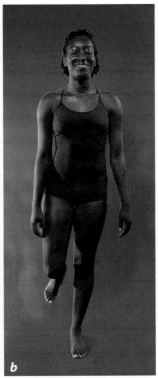
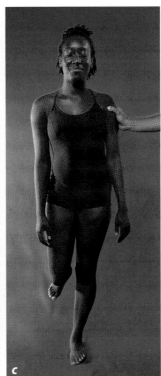
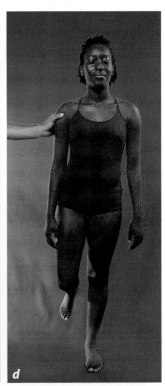

Figure 2.10   Proprioceptive exercises for the ankle. The athlete begins by balancing on one leg with *(a)* the eyes open and then *(b)* closed. *(c-d)* Increase the difficulty by applying a light force from an unknown direction. The athlete must contract the leg muscles to maintain balance.

ACHILLES TENDON STRAINS AND TENDINITIS

Running and jumping stress the Achilles tendon, the attachment of the gastrocnemius and soleus muscles to the heel. Achilles tendon **strains** and **tendinitis** are common athletic injuries. Older athletes and those who are infrequently physically active occasionally rupture this tendon completely.

Acute overstretching or a forceful contraction of the gastrocnemius and soleus muscles causes an Achilles tendon strain. Tendinitis tends to be an **overuse injury** that often occurs when athletes run or jump extensively. With either injury, the clinician should alleviate the athlete's discomfort by applying tape to limit excessive dorsiflexion.

Achilles Tendon Taping

Determine the amount of dorsiflexion that produces tendon discomfort. The athlete should

> **strain**—An overstretching (first degree), partial tearing (second degree), or complete rupture (third degree) of any component of the muscle-tendon unit.
>
> **tendinitis**—Inflammation of a tendon or its sheath.
>
> **overuse injury**—Chronic injury resulting from repetitive stress.

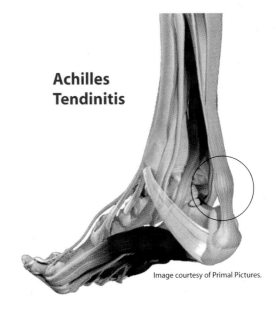

Achilles Tendinitis

Image courtesy of Primal Pictures.

slightly plantar flex and maintain this position during the procedure. The taping consists of applying anchors around the leg and foot and a series of strips to limit dorsiflexion. Elastic tape is the best material because it will guarantee that dorsiflexion will not come to an abrupt end. You may also supplement the taping procedure by inserting a 1/4-inch (0.6-centimeter) heel lift in *both* shoes (figure 2.11). When the athlete uses heel lifts, be certain that he or she regularly per-

forms stretching exercises to prevent adaptive shortening of the Achilles tendons.

Achilles Tendon Exercises

The exercises for the ankle are also appropriate for the Achilles tendon when the athlete gives special attention to stretching and strengthening the gastrocnemius and soleus muscles (see figures 2.8 and 2.9).

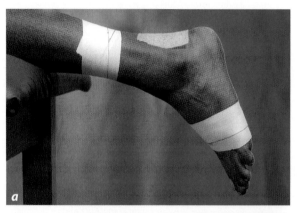

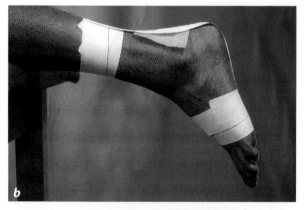

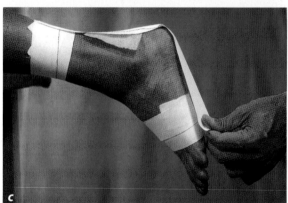

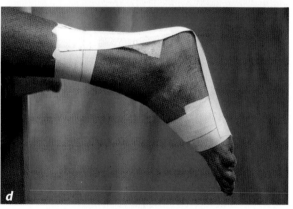

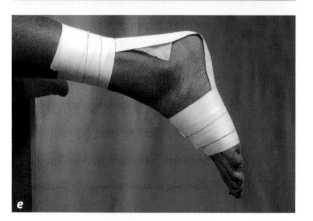

Figure 2.11 Taping procedure applied to limit extremes of dorsiflexion and, thus, to protect a strained or inflamed Achilles tendon. Identify the desired amount of dorsiflexion limitation and position the ankle accordingly. *(a)* Apply anchor strips proximally and distally with a friction pad to protect the Achilles tendon. *(b-d)* Supply three strips in an X fashion across the ankle to limit dorsiflexion. *(e)* Apply proximal and distal anchors.

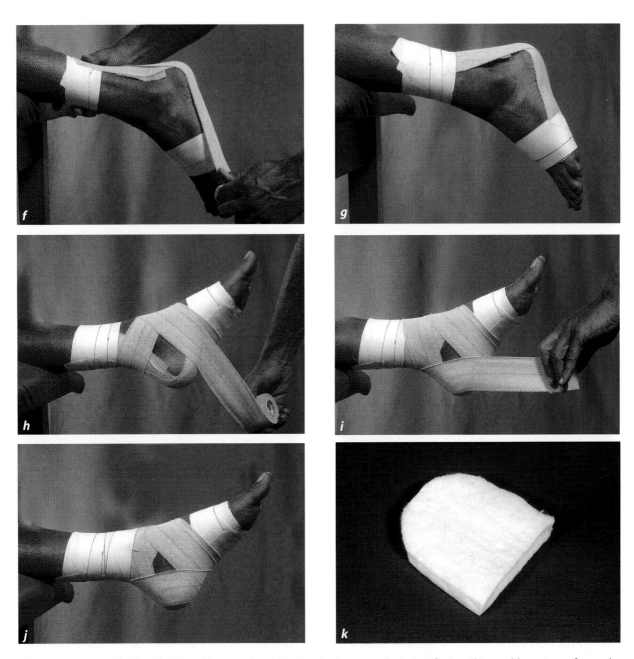

Figure 2.11 *(continued)* *(f-g)* Vary this procedure by using elastic tape to limit dorsiflexion. This would create a softer end point for limiting dorsiflexion. *(h-j)* Secure the entire procedure by applying both a figure eight and heel locks with elastic tape. *(k)* Supplement the procedure with a heel lift that can be placed in the athlete's shoe. Place the lift in both shoes to avoid creating a leg length discrepancy.

ARCH STRAINS AND PLANTAR FASCIITIS

Physically active people with a pes cavus foot experience strains to the arch or plantar fascia. Excessive running or jumping causes an arch strain. In addition, running, and particularly the continual stress that it places on the foot, precipitates **plantar fasciitis.** Poorly constructed and improperly fitted athletic footwear can also cause these injuries. Some athletes will experience relief from a commercially available plantar fasciitis brace (figure 2.12).

> **plantar fasciitis**—Inflammation of the plantar fascia at its attachment to the calcaneus.

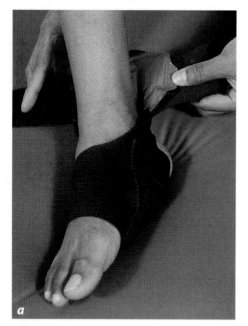

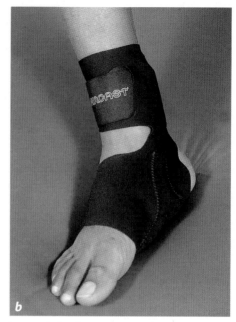

Figure 2.12   *(a-b)* A commercially produced brace that can help alleviate pain associated with plantar fasciitis.

Arch Taping

Support the longitudinal arch with a simple taping procedure (figure 2.13) or a more complex X-arch taping procedure (figure 2.14). The simple procedure employs three or four strips placed circularly around the foot. To complete an X-arch taping, place an anchor strip around the metatarsal heads and successively overlap strips from the anchor, around the heel, and back to the anchor.

A longitudinal arch pad may make this taping more efficacious (figure 2.15).

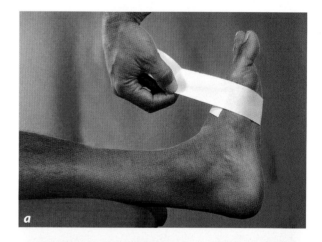

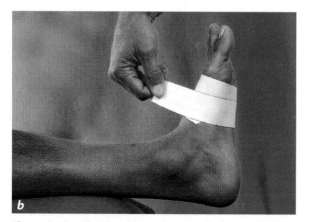

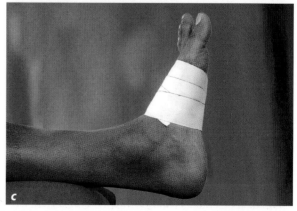

Figure 2.13   Simple taping to support the longitudinal arch. *(a-b)* Apply the tape by starting on the dorsum of the foot and then move in a lateral direction to lift, ultimately, the longitudinal arch. *(c)* Three or four strips will normally be adequate to support the longitudinal arch.

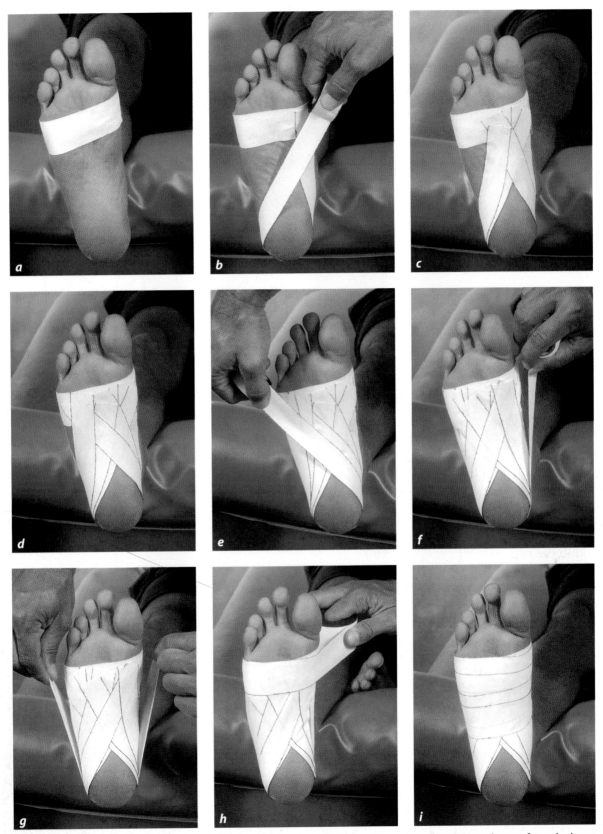

Figure 2.14 X-arch taping to support the longitudinal arch. *(a)* Following an anchor strip, *(b-c)* apply tape from the base of the great toe, around the heel, and back to the starting point. *(d)* Place subsequent strips from the medial to lateral aspect of the plantar surface of the foot. *(e-f)* Overlap strips from the lateral to medial aspect of the foot. *(g)* Apply a horseshoe strip from the lateral anchor to the medial anchor. *(h-i)* Complete the procedure with strips that mimic the simple arch taping procedure described in figure 2.13.

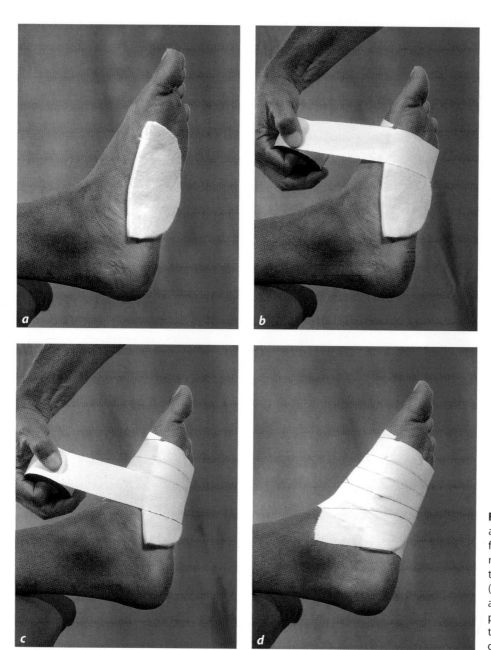

Figure 2.15 *(a)* Fashion a longitudinal arch pad from soft padding material and use it to support the athlete with a high (pes cavus) longitudinal arch. *(b-d)* Secure the arch pad to the foot using the simple arch taping described in figure 2.13.

Longitudinal Arch Exercises

Flexibility exercises should include stretching the gastrocnemius and soleus muscles (figure 2.8). Athletes can also stretch the arch by hyperextending the toes (figure 2.16).

Athletes can strengthen the arch by focusing on the intrinsic muscles of the foot. Activities such as picking up marbles with the toes and using toe curls to draw a towel across the floor will isolate these muscles (figure 2.17).

MORTON'S NEUROMA

This injury, also known as **plantar neuroma,** occurs when an interdigital nerve becomes inflamed where it passes between the heads of two metatarsal bones. Most often it affects the nerve between the third and fourth metatarsals, but it can involve other interdigital nerves. A

plantar neuroma—Inflammation or irritation of a plantar nerve.

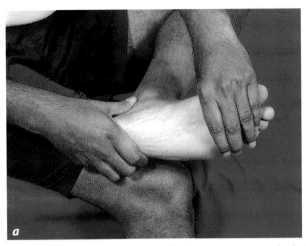
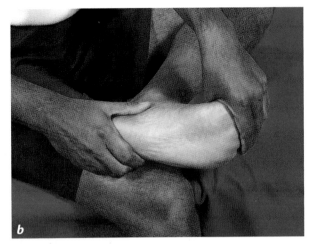

Figure 2.16   Stretch the plantar fascia by *(a)* grasping the ball of the foot and *(b)* extending the toes.

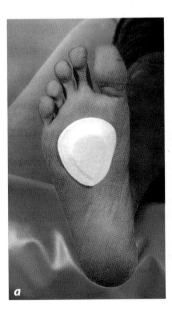

Figure 2.17   Strengthen the muscles that maintain the arch of the foot by curling a towel with the toes. As the muscles become stronger, add weight to the towel to provide muscle resistance.

fallen transverse arch or poor athletic footwear provides the mechanism for injury.

Transverse Arch Taping

Although athletic tape alone might provide adequate support for this injury, combining tape and a pad designed to support the transverse arch will be helpful. Use a commercially produced teardrop pad or a pad constructed from commercial padding and secure it in place with tape (figure 2.18). Completely resolving plantar neuroma may require more definitive medical treatment.

Transverse Arch Exercises

The longitudinal arch exercises may also be beneficial for this injury (see figures 2.16 and 2.17).

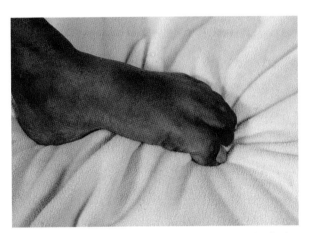
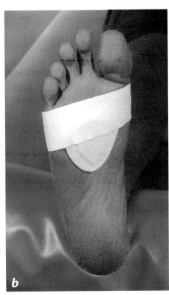
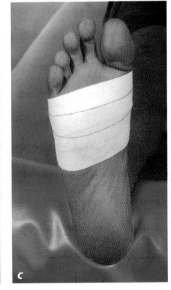

Figure 2.18 *(a)* Apply a commercially produced pad or cut a teardrop pad out of foam padding and *(b-c)* secure to the foot with tape. The tape should not be so tight that it restricts normal foot expansion during weight-bearing activity.

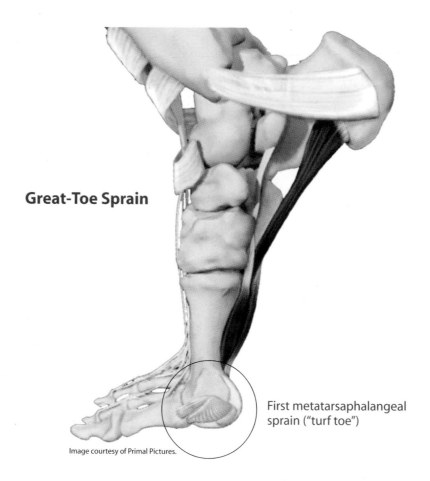

Great-Toe Sprain

First metatarsaphalangeal sprain ("turf toe")

Image courtesy of Primal Pictures.

GREAT-TOE SPRAINS

A sprain of the great toe, also known as turf toe, can be disabling. The injury usually results from hyperflexion or hyperextension of the first metatarsophalangeal joint. Athletes competing on artificial turf have a higher incidence of injury because of the enhanced shoe-ground interface.

Great-Toe Taping

Determine if hyperflexion or hyperextension produces the athlete's discomfort (figure 2.19). Begin the procedure by applying anchor strips around the midfoot and the great toe. Then, depending on the mechanism of injury, place longitudinal strips along the dorsal surface to

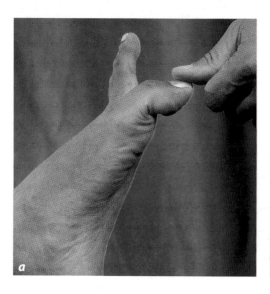
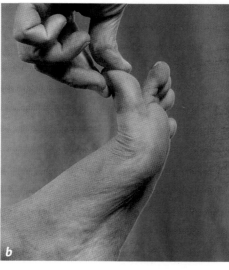

Figure 2.19
(a) Hyperflexion and *(b)* hyperextension of the great toe.

prevent hyperflexion or along the plantar surface to prevent hyperextension (figure 2.20). In some cases, strips of tape on both the dorsal and plantar surfaces may be necessary. Some athletes may prefer elastic tape for this procedure.

You may also purchase steel-plate inserts to use with the tape (figure 2.21).

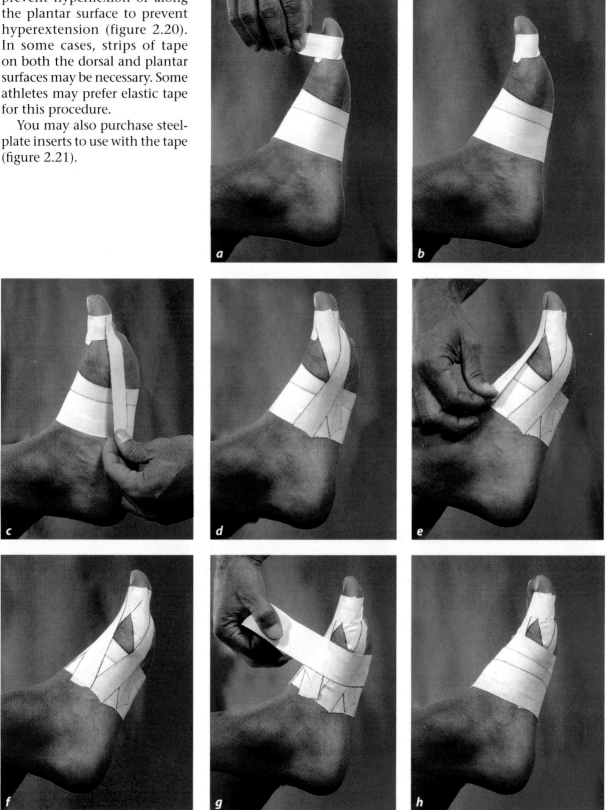

Figure 2.20   Taping for great-toe sprains, also known as turf toe. *(a-b)* Begin the procedure by applying anchor strips around the toe and foot. *(c-d)* Apply strips to the plantar surface of the foot to prevent hyperextension or *(e)* to both the plantar and dorsal surfaces of the foot to prevent hyperextension and hyperflexion. *(f)* Apply additional strips to provide extra support. *(g-h)* Complete the procedure by securing anchor strips around the toe and foot.

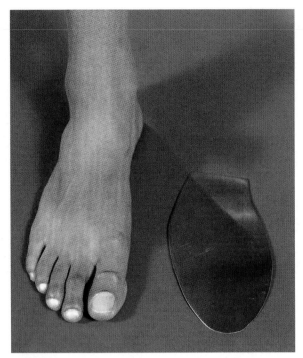

Figure 2.21 Use a steel-plate shoe insert to give additional support for turf toe by limiting flexion and extension of the great toe.

Great-Toe Exercises

The stretching and strengthening exercises for the longitudinal arch (see figures 2.16 and 2.17), when directed specifically to the great toe, will help the athlete recover from this injury.

HEEL CONTUSIONS

A thick fat pad protects the calcaneus, or heel bone, on the plantar surface of the foot. Nevertheless, contusions of the calcaneus often cause pain and disable a physically active person. Either acute trauma or chronic stress can precipitate this injury. Improper footwear can also bruise the heel.

Heel Contusion Taping

Figure 2.22 illustrates taping that supports the calcaneus. You can also secure a pad to the heel with basketweave taping.

SHIN SPLINTS

The colloquial term **shin splints** refers to leg pain that arises from a variety of sources, such as

arch strains, tendinitis, compartment syndrome, or stress fractures of the tibia or fibula. Seek the assistance of an experienced clinician to identify the source and mechanism of injury.

Arch Strains

A strain, or falling of the longitudinal arch, causes the tarsal bones of the foot to spread. The flattened foot can place undo stress where the extensor retinaculum ties the anterior tendons to the leg and cause the athlete to experience pain in the distal leg.

Tendinitis

Tendinitis may occur in any of the tendons that cross the ankle, but the posterior tibial tendon receives the greatest number of injuries. Running on uneven or banked surfaces that place one ankle in continuous eversion will precipitate injury. A hyperpronated foot could also contribute to the injury mechanism.

Compartment Syndrome

The tibia, fibula, and superficial fascia of the leg create a compartment through which the anterior muscles, the deep peroneal nerve, a vein, and an artery traverse. When the anterior muscles swell, they create chronic anterior compartment syndrome, producing leg pain and numbness that radiate into the foot.

Stress Fractures

Stress fractures to the tibia or fibula are a disruption to the **periosteum** and commonly occur in athletes who undergo prolonged periods of running. No taping procedure will help the symptoms associated with a stress fracture. The athlete usually requires 6 weeks of rest before the symptoms resolve.

shin splints—A colloquial term for pain in the leg that can originate from any number of possible sources.

periosteum—Outer layer of bone.

Shin Splint Taping

A haphazard taping approach often prevails in the treatment of shin splints. Several techniques exist

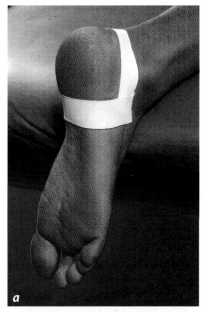

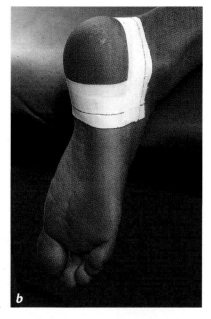

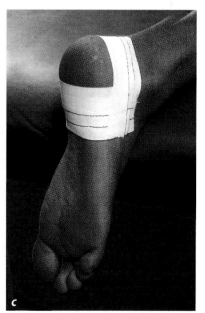

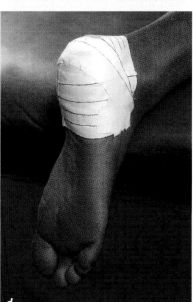

Figure 2.22 Support a bruised heel by applying tape designed to limit movement of the fat pad of the heel or to hold a protective pad in place. *(a)* Begin the procedure by applying anchor strips behind and below the heel. *(b-c)* Overlap strips in a weave pattern *(d)* until you completely cover the heel.

to remedy leg pain. If the pain occurs because of a fallen longitudinal arch, the athlete may find relief from simple arch taping combined with two or three strips placed around the distal leg to support the extensor retinaculum (figure 2.23). A closed basketweave designed to limit eversion aids posterior tibial tendinitis. Athletes have also reported relief from compression taping rather than from a procedure that supports the involved musculature (figure 2.24). No type of taping is likely to alleviate the effects of compartment syndrome or stress fractures.

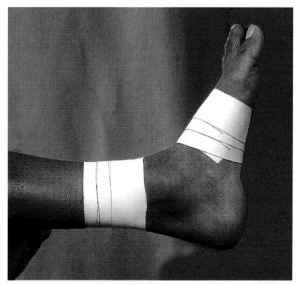

Figure 2.23 Taping procedure for shin splints caused by a weakened or fallen longitudinal arch. The procedure combines simple arch taping with reinforcement of the ankle retinacula. The retinacula secures the anterior tendons of the leg.

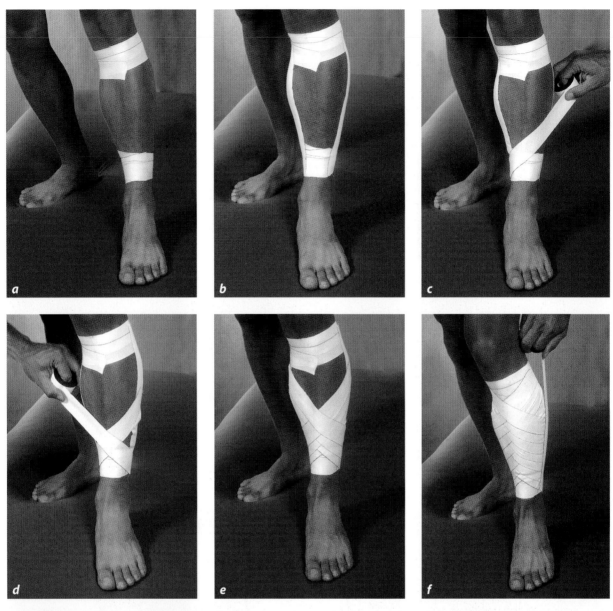

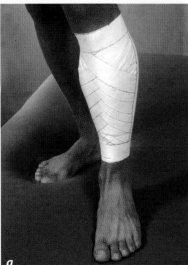

Figure 2.24   Apply tape to the anterior leg to support shin splints. Begin the procedure with (a) proximal and distal and (b) medial and lateral anchor strips. Apply tape in an oblique direction pulling (c) medial to lateral and (d) lateral to medial (e) in an overlapping fashion. Completely cover the anterior aspect of the leg. (f) Apply medial and lateral anchor strips (g) to complete the procedure.

Shin Splint Exercises

The stretching and strengthening exercises for the ankle (see figures 2.8 and 2.9) and longitudinal arch (see figures 2.16 and 2.17) can also be effective in decreasing leg pain. Have the athlete give special attention to achieving a balance between the strength of the anterior and posterior leg muscles. The athlete should also use high-quality footwear.

FOOT ORTHOTICS

Orthotics can treat many of the injuries described in this chapter. Figure 2.25 shows an **orthotic** that you can easily mold and send to the manufacturer for fabrication; other orthotics require a plaster cast. Prescribe orthotics wisely because they are expensive. Have an experienced clinician carefully evaluate the foot and lower-extremity biomechanics before recommending foot orthotics.

> **orthotic**—A commercially available insert designed to realign and alter the biomechanics of the foot.

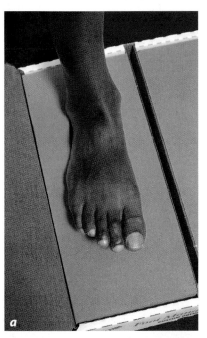

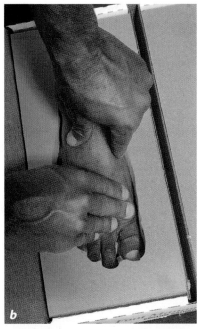

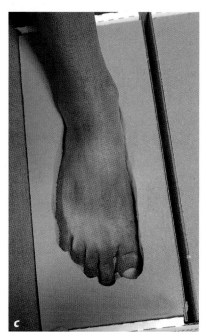

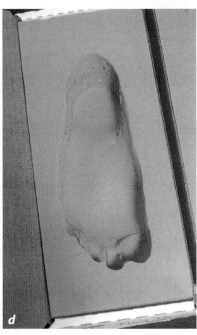

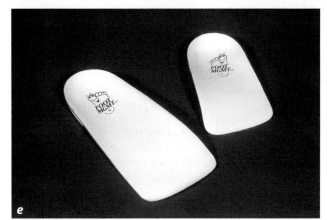

Figure 2.25   A foam imprint that will be used to produce an orthotic. *(a)* The athlete first pushes the heel to the bottom of the foam, and *(b)* then the athletic trainer pushes the forefoot and toes to the bottom of the foam *(c)* to make an imprint of the entire foot. *(d)* Send the impression to the manufacturer for fabrication of *(e)* the orthotic.

CHAPTER 3

The Knee

The articulation of the distal femur and the proximal tibia forms the knee. The proximal tibia and fibula also create a joint that you will find more relevant to normal ankle inversion and eversion than knee movement. The gliding action of the patella in the intercondylar fossa of the femur creates the patellofemoral articulation, a region essential to normal knee function.

Anterior Knee

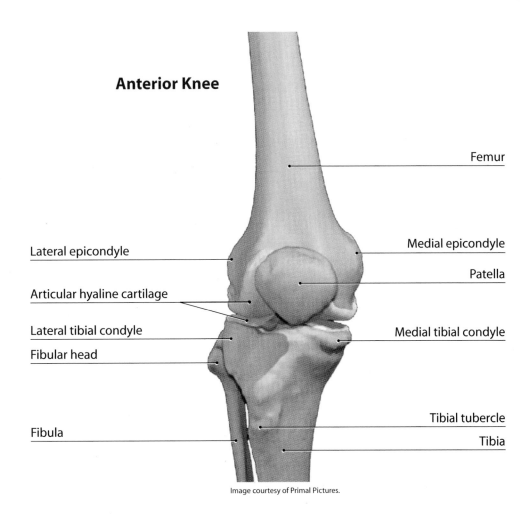

Lateral epicondyle	Femur
Articular hyaline cartilage	Medial epicondyle
Lateral tibial condyle	Patella
Fibular head	Medial tibial condyle
Fibula	Tibial tubercle
	Tibia

Image courtesy of Primal Pictures.

Knee movements include flexion and extension (figure 3.1). The knee is a modified hinge joint because the tibia internally rotates during flexion and externally rotates during extension.

Several ligaments stabilize the relatively shallow articulation between the femur and the tibia. The medial collateral ligament, also known as the tibial collateral ligament, supports the medial

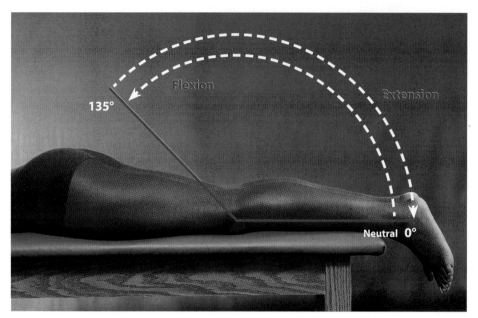

Figure 3.1   Knee flexion and extension ranges of motion.

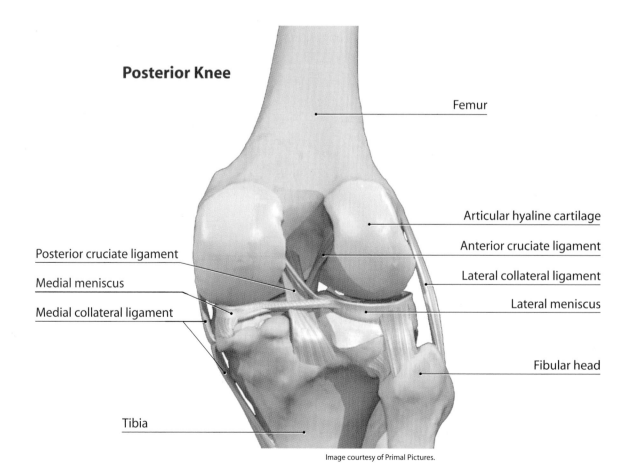

Image courtesy of Primal Pictures.

aspect of the knee by checking excess **valgus** displacement. The lateral collateral ligament, also called the fibular collateral ligament, stabilizes the lateral aspect of the knee by preventing excess **varus** displacement.

The anterior and posterior cruciate ligaments cross within the knee joint. The **anterior cruciate ligament** prevents the anterior displacement of the tibia from the femur; the posterior cruciate ligament checks posterior displacement. Because the cruciate ligaments prevent rotary instabilities, their injury frequently causes either anterior-lateral or anterior-medial rotary instability.

> **valgus**—Alignment of a joint or stress to the joint that places the distal bone in a lateral direction; the "knock-kneed" position of the knee joint.
>
> **varus**—Alignment of a joint or stress to the joint that places the distal bone in a medial direction; the "bow-legged" position of the knee joint.
>
> **anterior cruciate ligament**—A ligament crossing through the knee joint that attaches from the anterior tibia to the posterior femur. The anterior cruciate ligament limits anterior movement of the tibia from the femur as well as rotation of the tibia.

Anterior-lateral instability occurs when the lateral tibial condyle slips forward. Anterior-medial instability results when the medial tibial condyle slips forward. All these rotational instabilities disable physically active people.

The intra-articular cartilage, the **menisci**, deepens the articulation and protects the joint surfaces of the tibia and femur. The medial meniscus has an oval shape and firmly attaches to the tibia and the medial collateral ligament. In contrast, the lateral meniscus is more round and moves more freely; it does not attach to the lateral collateral ligament. Meniscal injuries are especially problematic because, as **avascular** cartilage, they rarely heal.

The knee extends through the contraction of the powerful **quadriceps femoris** muscles. These muscles include the rectus femoris, vastus medialis (see page 48), vastus intermedius, and vastus lateralis muscles. The fibers of the vastus

> **menisci**—The intra-articular cartilage of the knee.
>
> **avascular**—The absence of blood supply.
>
> **quadriceps femoris**—The muscle group in the anterior thigh consisting of the rectus femoris, vastus medialis, vastus intermedius, and vastus lateralis.

Knee Menisci

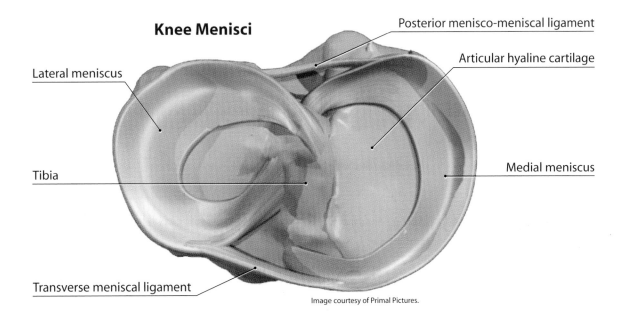

Lateral meniscus

Tibia

Transverse meniscal ligament

Posterior menisco-meniscal ligament

Articular hyaline cartilage

Medial meniscus

Image courtesy of Primal Pictures.

medialis muscle attach to the medial border of the patella, and they are often called the vastus medialis oblique muscle. The quadriceps attach to the patella through the tendon of the quadriceps; it passes over and around the patella and attaches to the tibia as the patellar tendon. These muscles suffer contusions during the athlete's participation in contact sports.

The **hamstring** muscle group produces knee flexion. These muscles include the medial semitendinosus and semimembranosus and the lateral biceps femoris; all these muscles experience strain during sprinting activities.

Several bursae exist around the knee to reduce the friction that the overlying muscle tendons create. These **bursae** include the suprapatellar, prepatellar, and the deep and superficial infrapatellar bursae. The suprapatellar directly communicates with the capsule of the knee joint. Excess fluid in this bursa represents significant swelling in the knee. The prepatellar bursa has a high contusion rate because of its anterior position to the joint.

hamstrings—A muscle group in the posterior thigh consisting of the semitendinosus, semimembranosus, and biceps femoris.

bursa—A fluid sac that reduces friction between two structures.

Anterior Thigh Muscles

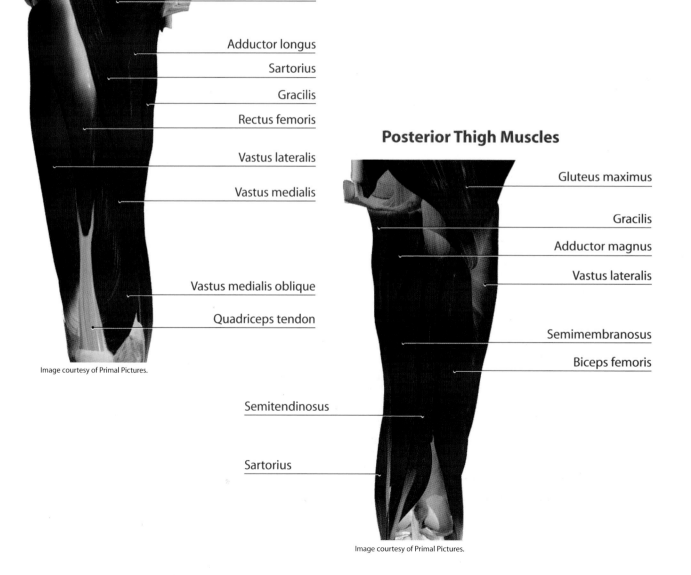

Pectineus

Adductor longus

Sartorius

Gracilis

Rectus femoris

Vastus lateralis

Vastus medialis

Vastus medialis oblique

Quadriceps tendon

Image courtesy of Primal Pictures.

Posterior Thigh Muscles

Gluteus maximus

Gracilis

Adductor magnus

Vastus lateralis

Semimembranosus

Biceps femoris

Semitendinosus

Sartorius

Image courtesy of Primal Pictures.

Key Palpation Landmarks

Medial Aspect	**Lateral Aspect**	**Anterior Aspect**	**Posterior Aspect**
▸ Medial collateral ligament	▸ Lateral collateral ligament	▸ Quadriceps tendon	▸ Popliteal fossa
▸ Medial joint line	▸ Lateral joint line	▸ Patella	▸ Biceps femoris tendon
▸ Medial meniscus	▸ Lateral meniscus	▸ Patellar tendon	▸ Semitendinosus tendon
			▸ Semimembranosus tendon

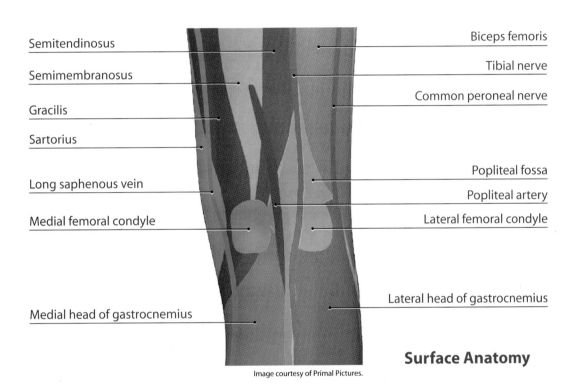

Semitendinosus

Semimembranosus

Gracilis

Sartorius

Long saphenous vein

Medial femoral condyle

Medial head of gastrocnemius

Biceps femoris

Tibial nerve

Common peroneal nerve

Popliteal fossa

Popliteal artery

Lateral femoral condyle

Lateral head of gastrocnemius

Surface Anatomy

Image courtesy of Primal Pictures.

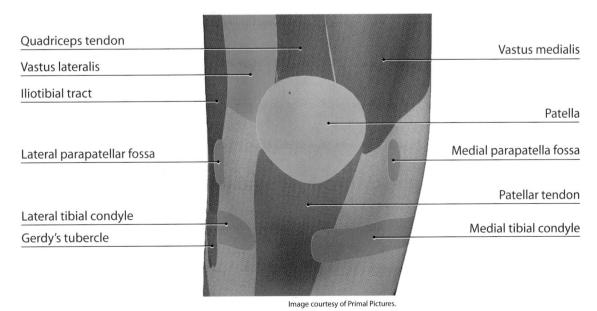

Quadriceps tendon

Vastus lateralis

Iliotibial tract

Lateral parapatellar fossa

Lateral tibial condyle

Gerdy's tubercle

Vastus medialis

Patella

Medial parapatella fossa

Patellar tendon

Medial tibial condyle

Image courtesy of Primal Pictures.

COLLATERAL AND CRUCIATE LIGAMENT SPRAINS

The relative instability of the knee renders it highly vulnerable to sprains of the collateral and cruciate ligaments. Excessive valgus or varus forces sprain the medial and lateral collateral ligaments, respectively. You can expect to see fewer injuries to the lateral collateral ligament because the **contralateral** extremity protects the knee from varus forces. External forces directed at the outside of the knee produce valgus stress; they often implicate the anterior cruciate ligament and medial meniscus as well as the medial collateral ligament. Clinicians refer to this classic injury as the terrible triad.

contralateral—Refers to the opposite extremity.

Noncontact mechanisms often cause isolated injuries to the cruciate ligaments, particularly the anterior cruciate. Sudden deceleration, which occurs when the athlete changes direction or dismounts from a gymnastic apparatus, can produce an isolated rupture of the anterior cruciate ligament. An external force anteriorly directed to the back of the tibia will also injure the anterior cruciate ligament, just as a posteriorly directed force from the front of the knee can injure the posterior cruciate ligament.

Anterior Cruciate Ligament Rupture

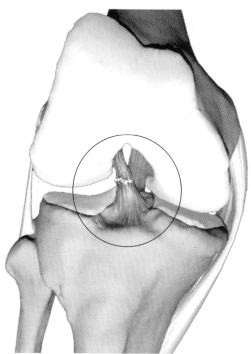

Image courtesy of Primal Pictures.

Medial Collateral Ligament Rupture

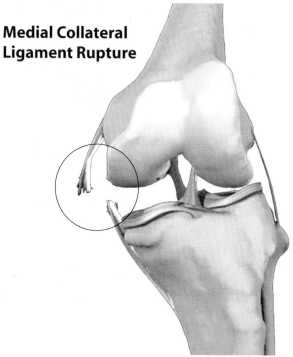

Image courtesy of Primal Pictures.

Knee Sprain Taping

Figure 3.2 illustrates how to tape the collateral ligaments. Execute a slight flexion by placing a lift under the heel. Avoid using a tape roll for this lift because heel pressure will ruin the tape! As with the ankle, optimize the procedure by taping directly on shaved skin and using minimal underwrap. I recommend elastic tape. Begin by placing proximal and distal anchors and then apply, in an X pattern, successive interlocking strips over the medial and lateral collateral ligaments. For the athlete with a cruciate ligament injury, tape a series of medial and lateral spiral strips to enhance anterior, posterior, and rotary support.

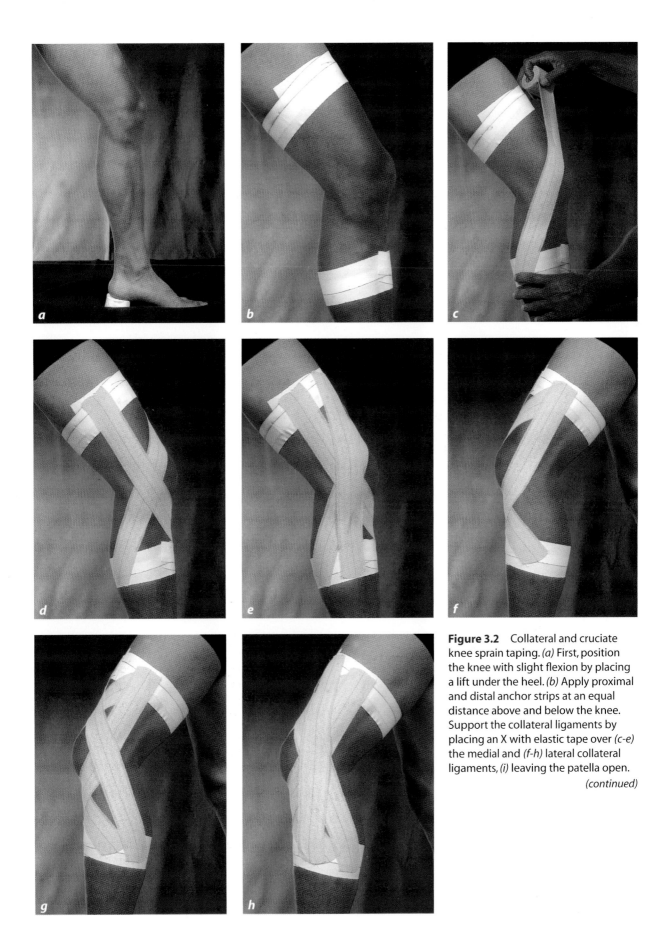

Figure 3.2 Collateral and cruciate knee sprain taping. *(a)* First, position the knee with slight flexion by placing a lift under the heel. *(b)* Apply proximal and distal anchor strips at an equal distance above and below the knee. Support the collateral ligaments by placing an X with elastic tape over *(c-e)* the medial and *(f-h)* lateral collateral ligaments, *(i)* leaving the patella open.

(continued)

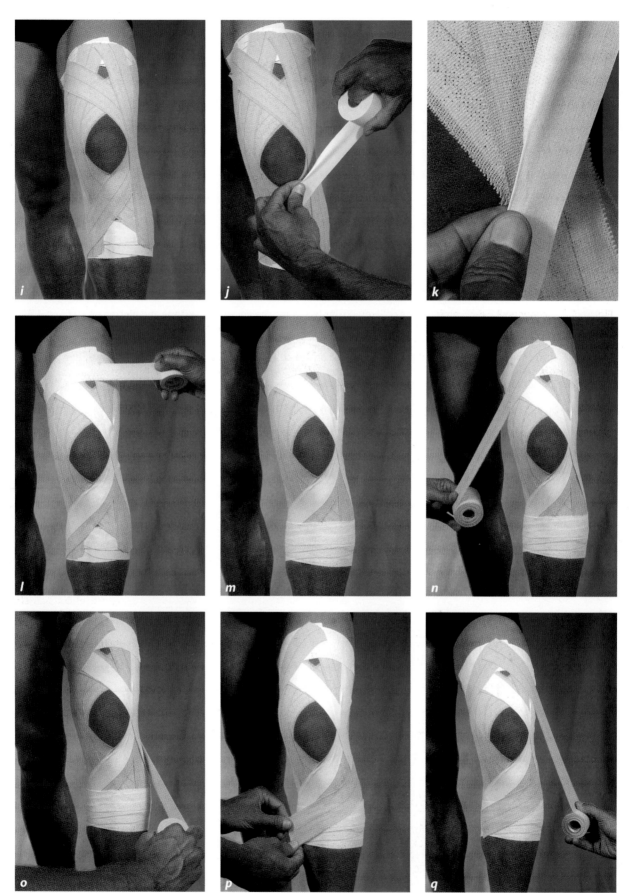

Figure 3.2 *(continued)*

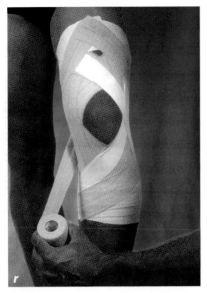
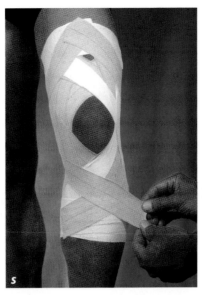
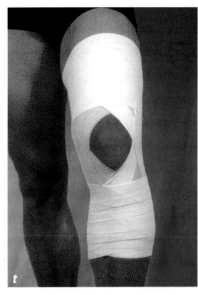

Figure 3.2   *(continued)*   *(j-k)* Reinforce the collateral strips by folding the edge of white tape and placing an additional X over the previously applied elastic tape. *(l-m)* Apply proximal and distal anchors to complete the collateral knee sprain taping. *(n-s)* For rotary instability that often results from injury to the anterior cruciate ligament, apply additional strips that begin on the anterior-proximal thigh, pass behind the knee, and end on the posterior leg. *(t)* Complete the procedure by enclosing the thigh and leg with elastic tape.

Knee Exercises

Injury-free, effective athletic participation requires the quadriceps and hamstring muscles to have adequate strength and flexibility. Figure 3.3 illustrates static stretching exercises for these groups.

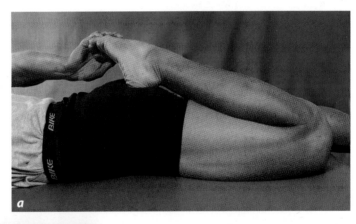

Figure 3.3   *(a)* Stretch the quadriceps muscle group by pulling the knee into flexion while the athlete is lying prone. *(b)* Stretch the hamstring by flexing the hip while maintaining knee extension. Note how the athlete holds the back in a flattened position to ensure optimal isolation of the hamstring muscles.

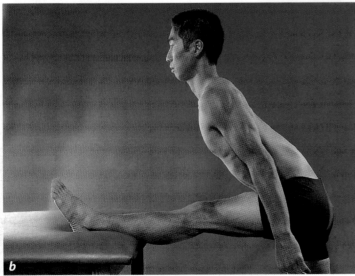

Strengthen the athlete's quadriceps and hamstring muscles by prescribing **open-chain exercises** with elastic bands (figure 3.4).

Figure 3.5 illustrates a strengthening device that provides progressive resistance for the knee.

Weight-bearing exercises from closed-chain positions will build the athlete's strength and functional ability. The step-up (figure 3.6) and squat exercises (figure 3.7) are simple, yet effective, **closed-chain exercises.**

open-chain exercise—Exercise in which the distal segment of the extremity does not bear weight.

closed-chain exercise—Exercise in which the distal segment of the extremity is fixed to the ground.

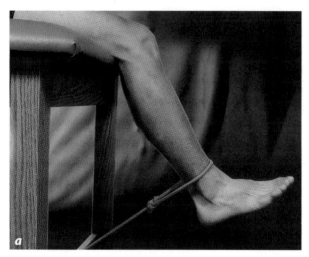

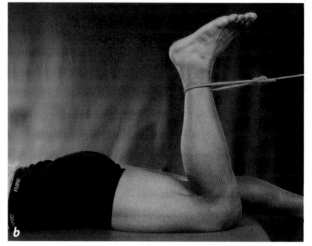

Figure 3.4 *(a)* Strengthen the quadriceps by resisting knee extension while the athlete is seated. *(b)* Strengthen the hamstring muscle group by providing resistance to knee flexion while the athlete is lying prone.

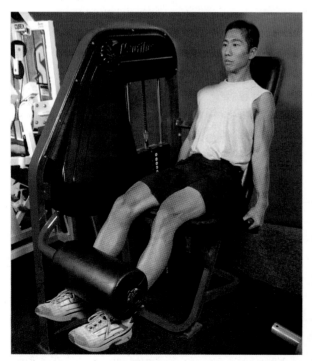

Figure 3.5 Strengthen the quadriceps and hamstring muscles with a commercially available resistance device.

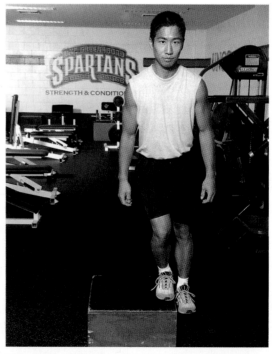

Figure 3.6 The step-up is an excellent example of a closed-chain exercise that incorporates the quadriceps as a knee extensor and the hamstrings as a hip extensor.

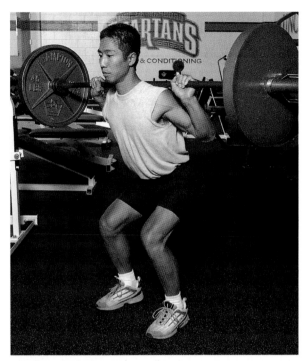

Figure 3.7   Closed-chain squat exercise for the knee extensor and hip extensor muscles.

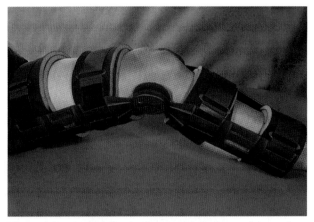

Figure 3.8   A rehabilitative brace with flexion and extension stops that can be used to control the degree of knee motion.

KNEE BRACES

Knee braces fall into three categories: preventive, rehabilitative, and functional.

Preventive Braces

Preventive braces guard the knee from injury during athletic participation by protecting the medial collateral ligament from excessive valgus force. Speculation abounds concerning the potential of this brace to reduce injury to the medial collateral ligament, and they are used far less frequently than they were in the past. Although athletes, coaches, and athletic trainers offer anecdotal reports that the brace has saved the ligament, scientific research is less conclusive on the value of the preventive knee brace. I am wary of prescribing a preventive device because of its questionable clinical value and excessive cost.

Rehabilitative Braces

Rehabilitative braces protect the knee immediately after injury or surgery (figure 3.8). Clinicians can control the range of motion of the knee by adjusting dials on the medial and lateral aspects of the brace.

Functional Braces

Functional knee braces may be used on athletes who experience rotary instability because of injury to the anterior cruciate ligament (figures 3.9 and 3.10). Some physicians recommend or require a functional brace following surgical reconstruction of a knee with a deficient anterior cruciate ligament. Athletes have found functional knee braces effective for some anterior cruciate ligament injuries; others require surgical reconstruction before returning to competition. The functional knee brace has the disadvantage of costing at least several hundred dollars.

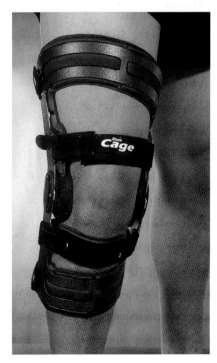

Figure 3.9   A functional knee brace to control rotary instability of the knee.

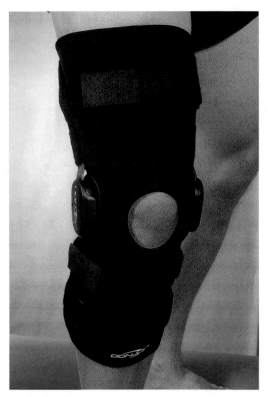

Figure 3.10 A functional knee brace with flexion and extension stops that can also control the amount of knee motion.

KNEE HYPEREXTENSION

Knee hyperextension occurs when an anteriorly directed or self-inflicted force causes the joint to extend beyond its normal anatomical limits. The cruciate ligaments, as well as the muscles and capsule located on the posterior aspect of the knee, may suffer damage.

Hyperextension Taping

Determine the degree of extension required to elicit knee discomfort. Place a lift under the heel to flex the athlete's joint slightly. Be certain that the athlete maintains this position for the entire procedure. Begin by placing anchor strips around the thigh and calf and then supply successive strips in an X-pattern from the proximal to distal anchors over the posterior aspect of the joint. You may wish to complete the taping procedure by using an elastic wrap to enclose the knee (figure 3.11).

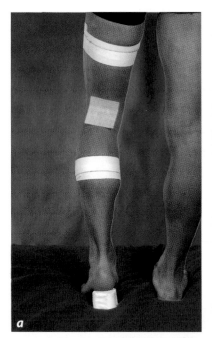
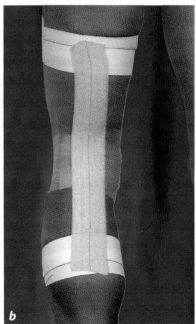
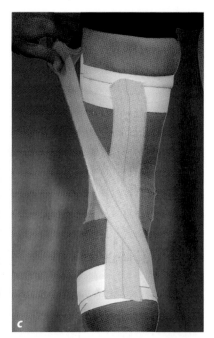

Figure 3.11 Begin knee hyperextension taping by placing a lift under the heel to flex the knee. *(a)* Protect the back of the knee with a pad and apply proximal and distal anchor strips. *(b)* Use elastic tape to apply a vertical strip and *(c-e)* then overlap with two strips, creating an X over the back of the knee. *(f)* Apply proximal and distal anchors to secure the procedure. *(g-h)* Complete the procedure by enclosing the knee in an elastic wrap.

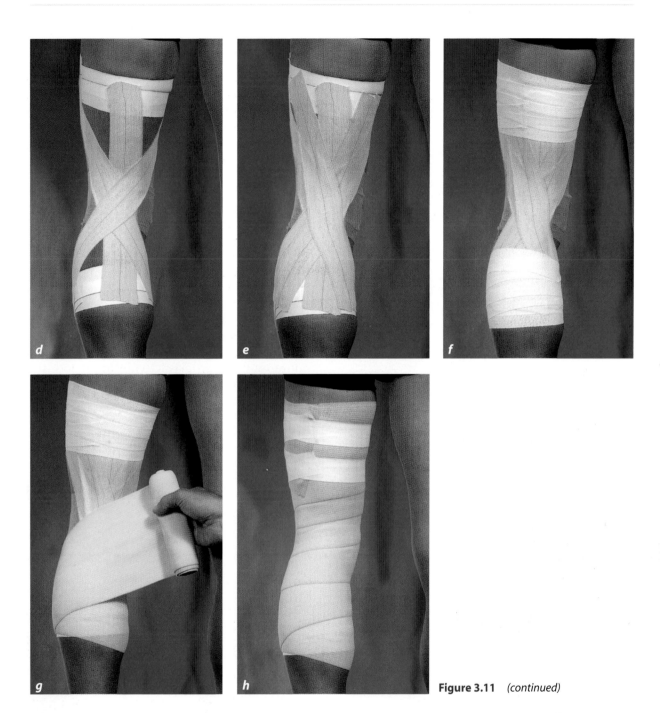

Figure 3.11   *(continued)*

Hyperextension Exercises

Exercise should restore normal flexibility and strength of the hamstring. The stretching and strengthening exercises for knee sprains (see figures 3.3 and 3.4) will accomplish this goal.

PATELLOFEMORAL JOINT PAIN

Physically active people commonly experience extensor mechanism pain arising from the patellofemoral articulation. Because this pain may result from numerous causes, an experienced clinician should carefully analyze the athlete's condition. The injury mechanisms include a malalignment of the patella, an increased **quadriceps (q)-angle,** hyperpronation of the feet, or a weak vastus medialis oblique muscle.

quadriceps (q)-angle—The degree of obliquity of the quadriceps.

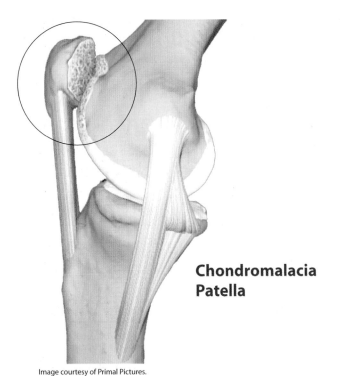

Chondromalacia Patella

Image courtesy of Primal Pictures.

Patellofemoral Taping

Provide patellofemoral support to displace the patella medially or realign it. Knee sleeves with lateral buttresses will supply medial displacement (figure 3.12), and the McConnel taping technique will realign the patella (figure 3.13). The taping procedure requires you to evaluate both the position of the patella and the patient's response to your treatment. Carefully analyze whether the taping relieves the athlete's pain while he or she performs functional activities. McConnel taping, which requires a special tape more rigid than the nonelastic variety, is only one component of a complete patellofemoral treatment and rehabilitation program.

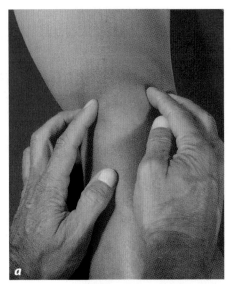

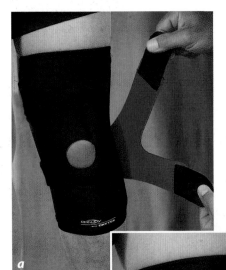

Figure 3.12 *(a-b)* Use a knee sleeve with a lateral buttress to facilitate normal tracking of the patella within the intercondylar fossa of the femur.

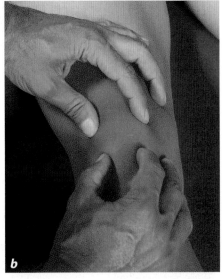

Figure 3.13 McConnel taping for an athlete with patellofemoral pain. *(a-b)* Assess the patella for tilt and rotation positioning.

(continued)

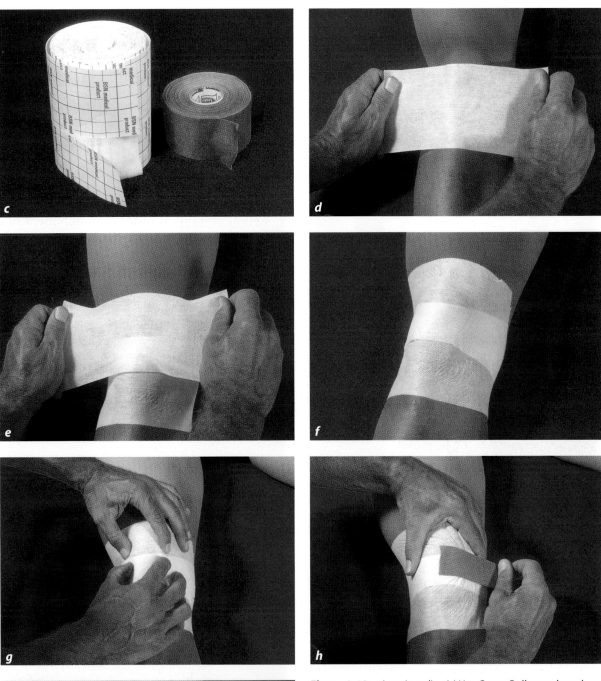

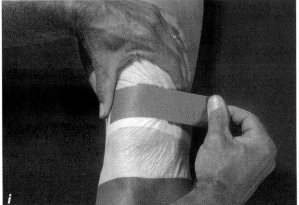

Figure 3.13 *(continued)* *(c)* Use Cover-Roll stretch and Leukotape (available from Beiersdorf Inc., P.O. Box 5529, Norwalk, CT 06856-5529) for the taping procedure. *(d-f)* After shaving the knee, cover the patella with Cover-Roll tape and *(g)* then reassess for position. *(h)* Correct tilt of the patella by applying a piece of Leukotape from the middle of the patella to the medial femoral condyle. *(i)* Correct glide of the patella by applying the Leukotape from the lateral border of the patella and pulling medially to the medial femoral condyle.

(continued)

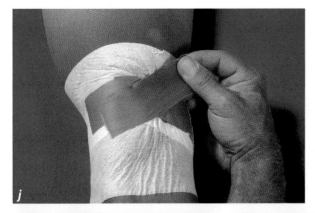

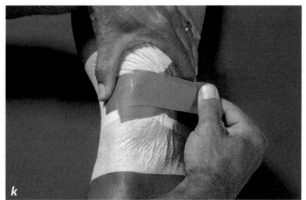

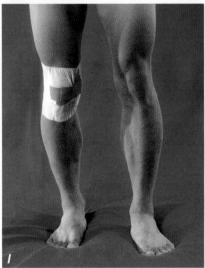

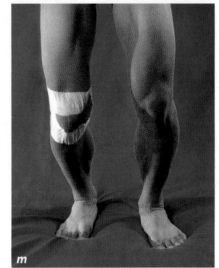

Figure 3.13   *(continued)*
(j) Correct external rotation by applying Leukotape from the inferior pole (border) of the patella, pulling toward the opposite shoulder. *(k)* If the tilt of the patella is not correct, apply an additional tilt strip. *(l-m)* Reassess the athlete for pain while he or she performs the functional activities that cause discomfort.

Extensor Mechanism Exercises

The stretching exercises for knee sprains, which restore the normal flexibility of both the quadriceps and hamstring muscles, will also help athletes who experience patellofemoral pain. The athlete should also strengthen the quadriceps muscles, although providing resistance to knee extension through the full range of motion of the joint may increase patellofemoral compression and aggravate the injury. Modify the quadriceps strengthening exercises for knee sprains to isolate the extension of the knee in its final 30° or find the range of motion through which the athlete can exercise pain-free. Although not as effective as resisted knee extension, straight-leg raises will also exercise the quadriceps without significantly increasing patellofemoral compression (figure 3.14). If necessary, use **electrical muscle stimulation** or **biofeedback** to strengthen the vastus medialis oblique muscle—techniques that you will learn in your therapeutic exercise class.

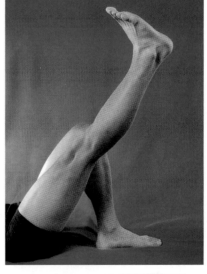

Figure 3.14
Use straight-leg raises to strengthen the muscles of the quadriceps without concomitant increases in patellofemoral compression.

electrical muscle stimulation—Use of electrical current to induce a muscle to contract.

biofeedback—Feedback provided through visual observation or an audio tone.

CHAPTER 4

The Thigh, Hip, and Pelvis

The ball of the hip, the head of the femur, the socket, and the acetabulum of the pelvis create an extremely stable articulation.

The pelvic girdle contains two **innominate bones,** each possessing an ilium, a pubis, and an ischium. The pelvis protects the abdomen and joins many of the muscles acting on the hip and trunk.

innominate bones—Two flat bones that form the pelvic girdle; each consists of an ilium, pubis, and ischium.

Anterior Hip and Pelvis

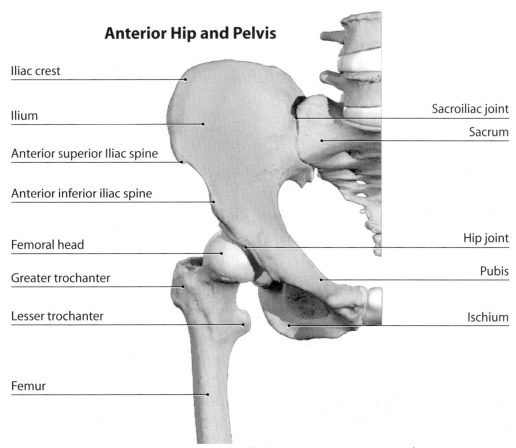

Iliac crest

Ilium

Anterior superior Iliac spine

Anterior inferior iliac spine

Femoral head

Greater trochanter

Lesser trochanter

Femur

Sacroiliac joint

Sacrum

Hip joint

Pubis

Ischium

Image courtesy of Primal Pictures.

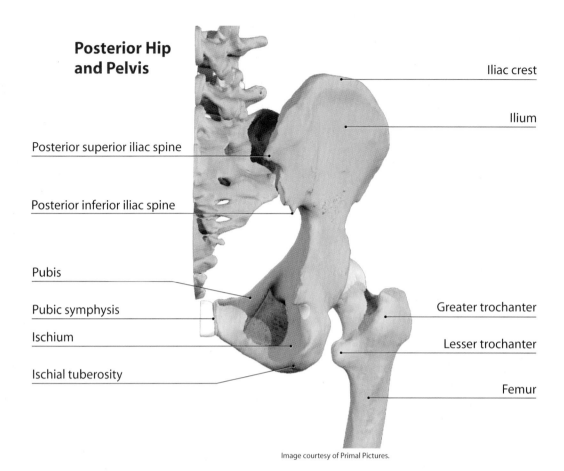

Posterior Hip and Pelvis

Iliac crest

Ilium

Posterior superior iliac spine

Posterior inferior iliac spine

Pubis

Pubic symphysis

Ischium

Ischial tuberosity

Greater trochanter

Lesser trochanter

Femur

Image courtesy of Primal Pictures.

Hip joint movements include flexion and extension, abduction and adduction, medial and lateral rotation (figure 4.1), and **circumduction.**

circumduction—A combination of abduction, adduction, flexion, and extension.

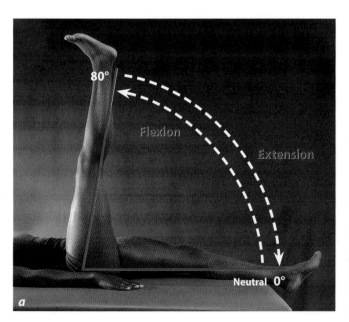

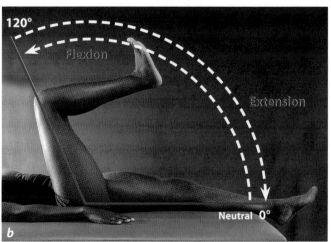

Figure 4.1 Hip flexion and extension ranges of motion with *(a)* knee extended and *(b)* flexed; *(continued)*

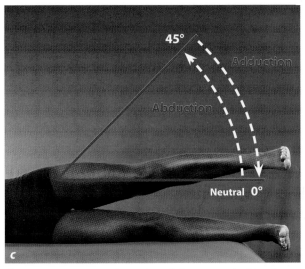

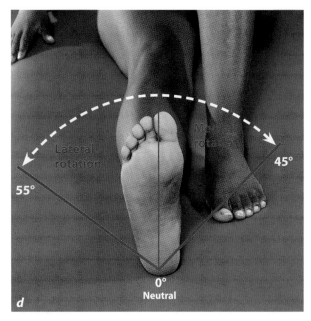

Figure 4.1 *(continued)* *(c)* hip abduction and adduction ranges of motion; *(d)* hip medial and lateral rotation ranges of motion.

A thick capsule and three major ligaments reinforce the hip joint. The anterior ligament, called the Y-ligament, is the iliofemoral; it checks excessive hip extension. The medial ligament, also known as the pubofemoral ligament, limits excess hip abduction. The ischiofemoral ligament, located on the posterior, becomes taut during hip flexion.

The depth of the hip joint, combined with its substantial capsular and ligament structures, contributes to the considerable stability of this joint.

Several muscle groups govern movement at this multidirectional joint. The iliopsoas and the rectus femoris muscles of the quadriceps produce flexion. Extension results from the contraction

Hip Ligaments

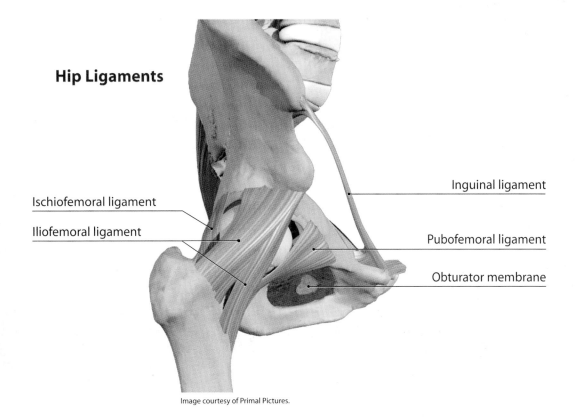

Ischiofemoral ligament

Iliofemoral ligament

Inguinal ligament

Pubofemoral ligament

Obturator membrane

Image courtesy of Primal Pictures.

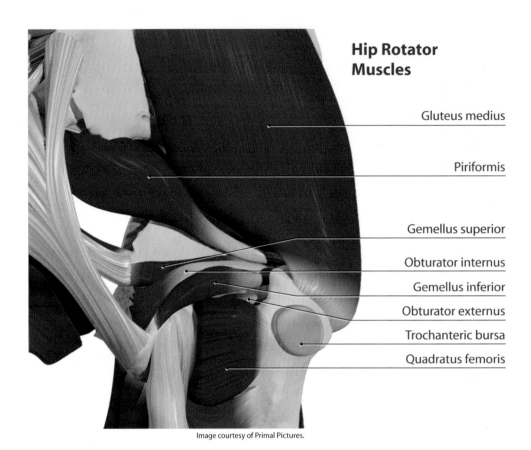

Hip Rotator Muscles

Gluteus medius

Piriformis

Gemellus superior

Obturator internus

Gemellus inferior

Obturator externus

Trochanteric bursa

Quadratus femoris

Image courtesy of Primal Pictures.

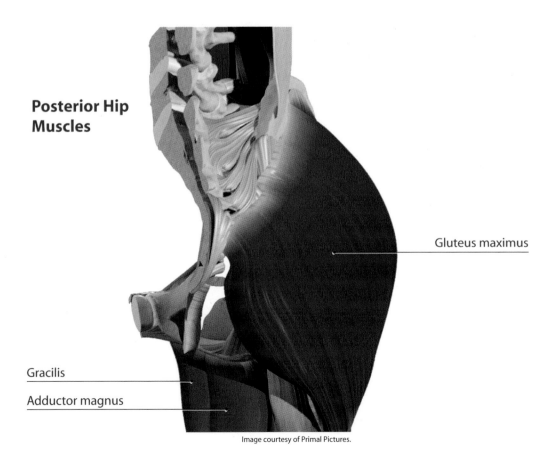

Posterior Hip Muscles

Gluteus maximus

Gracilis

Adductor magnus

Image courtesy of Primal Pictures.

of the gluteus maximus and the three hamstring muscles.

The gluteus medius and tensor fasciae latae muscles produce primary abduction, and the adductor magnus, longus, and brevis muscles cause adduction. The muscle group that includes the piriformis, gemellus superior and inferior, obturator internus and externus, and the quadratus femoris produces outward rotation. The tensor fasciae latae produces inward rotation.

HIP STRAINS

Hip muscle strains, or groin pulls, involve either the hip flexor muscles or the adductor muscle group. The athlete usually overstretches or violently contracts the muscles. Lack of flexibility or strength, as well as inadequate preexercise warm-up, will precipitate strains.

Key Palpation Landmarks

Anterior

- ▸ Rectus femoris muscle
- ▸ Vastus medialis muscle
- ▸ Vastus lateralis muscle
- ▸ Anterior superior iliac spine

Medial

- ▸ Adductor longus muscle
- ▸ Gracilis muscle
- ▸ Adductor magnus muscle

Lateral

- ▸ Iliac crest

Posterior

- ▸ Posterior superior iliac spine
- ▸ Ischial tuberosity
- ▸ Gluteus maximus muscle
- ▸ Biceps femoris muscle
- ▸ Semitendinosus muscle
- ▸ Semimembranosus muscle

Surface Anatomy

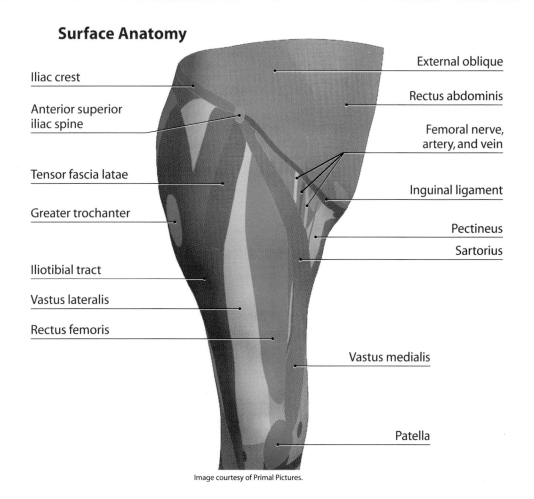

Iliac crest

Anterior superior iliac spine

Tensor fascia latae

Greater trochanter

Iliotibial tract

Vastus lateralis

Rectus femoris

External oblique

Rectus abdominis

Femoral nerve, artery, and vein

Inguinal ligament

Pectineus

Sartorius

Vastus medialis

Patella

Image courtesy of Primal Pictures.

Hip Strain Taping

Support the hip muscles with an elastic bandage supplemented with elastic tape. Wrap the bandage around the thigh and hip in a **spica** pattern. Before treatment you should determine if the athlete has damaged the hip flexor or adductor muscles. Examine for pain or weakness in these groups by using resistance to test hip flexion and adduction, in that order (figure 4.2). The affected muscle group will determine the direction in which you apply the hip spica.

spica—A figure-eight wrap that incorporates the thigh and hip or the arm and shoulder.

When wrapping adductor muscles, have the athlete internally rotate the hip. Place the wrap from a lateral to medial direction. Begin at midthigh and proceed to encircle the thigh and wind around the waist (figure 4.3). Use double-length elastic wrap, if available, and reinforce the wrap by tracing the pattern with elastic tape.

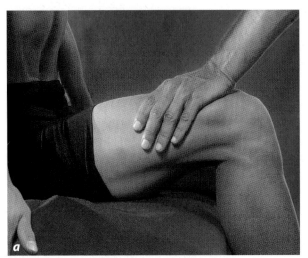
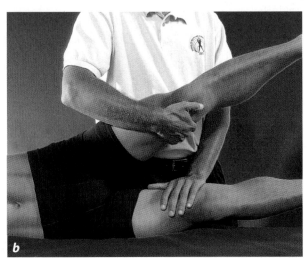

Figure 4.2   *(a)* Test the hip flexor muscles for strength by resisting the athlete's efforts to flex the hip while seated. *(b)* Test the adductor muscles by having the athlete on his or her side. The athlete then resists your efforts to abduct the right extremity.

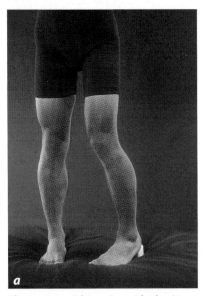
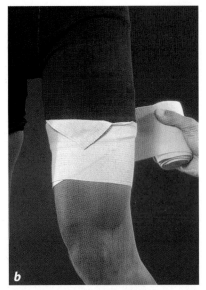
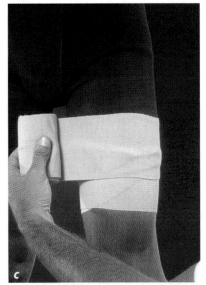

Figure 4.3   A hip spica with elastic wrap to support a strain of the adductor muscles. *(a)* Have the athlete place the hip in an internally rotated position. *(b-c)* Apply an elastic wrap by pulling the thigh into internal rotation. Note how the elastic wrap folds over itself to lock it in place.   *(continued)*

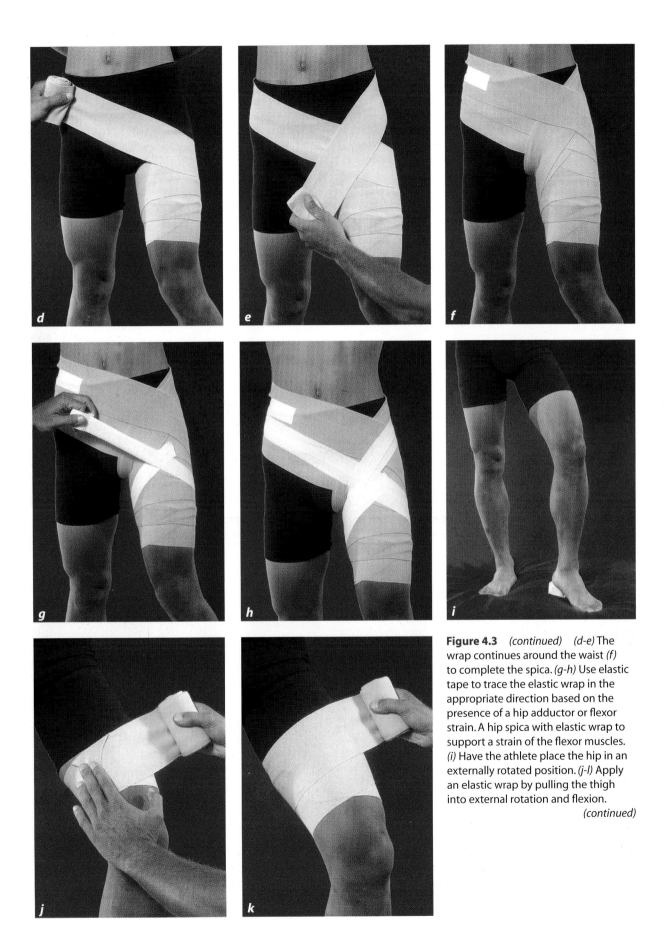

Figure 4.3 *(continued)* *(d-e)* The wrap continues around the waist *(f)* to complete the spica. *(g-h)* Use elastic tape to trace the elastic wrap in the appropriate direction based on the presence of a hip adductor or flexor strain. A hip spica with elastic wrap to support a strain of the flexor muscles. *(i)* Have the athlete place the hip in an externally rotated position. *(j-l)* Apply an elastic wrap by pulling the thigh into external rotation and flexion.

(continued)

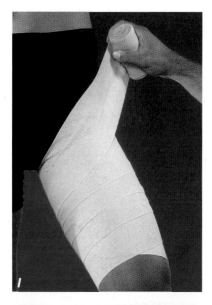

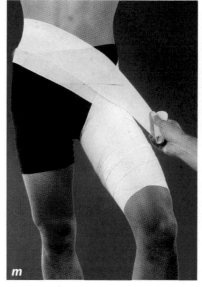

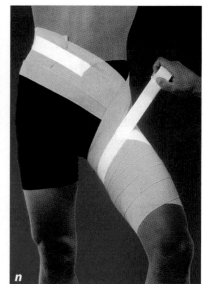

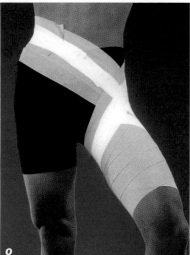

Figure 4.3 *(continued)* *(m)* The wrap continues around the waist to complete the spica. *(n-o)* Use elastic tape to trace the elastic wrap in the same direction as the elastic wrap.

Use a similar procedure to support the hip flexor muscles, except begin with the hip in an externally rotated position and reverse the direction of the pull of the wrap. Before applying the wrap, place a lift under the heel of the extremity to shorten the hip flexors.

Hip Exercises

The athlete must maintain normal strength and flexibility in the hip muscles to prevent or treat strains. Figure 4.4 illustrates a static stretching exercise for the hip. Elastic bands can also supply resistance to strengthen the joint (figure 4.5). Because the rectus femoris of the quadriceps and all three hamstring muscles act on the hip, the exercises for these groups are also appropriate (see chapter 3).

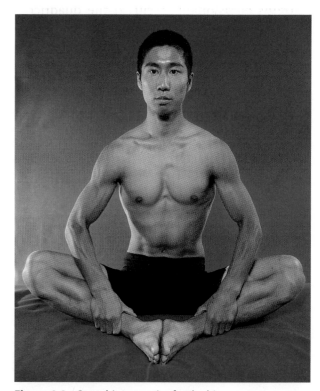

Figure 4.4 Stretching exercise for the hip.

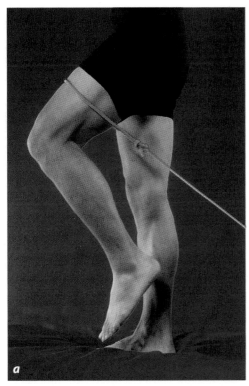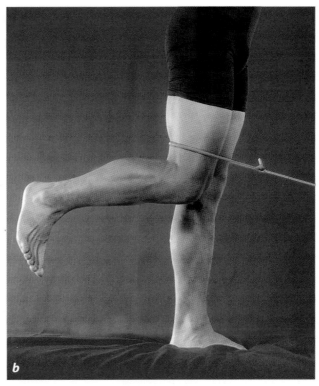

Figure 4.5 Strengthening exercises for *(a)* the hip flexor and *(b)* extensor muscles.

THIGH STRAINS

Strains occasionally occur to the quadriceps femoris muscles and more frequently to the hamstrings. The strain may result from overstretching, a violent contraction, or general muscle fatigue. For hamstring strains, determine whether the injury involves the medial (semitendinosus and semimembranosus) or the lateral (biceps femoris) muscles. Isolate the medial and lateral hamstrings during muscle testing by rotating the leg internally and externally, respectively, during resisted knee flexion (figure 4.6).

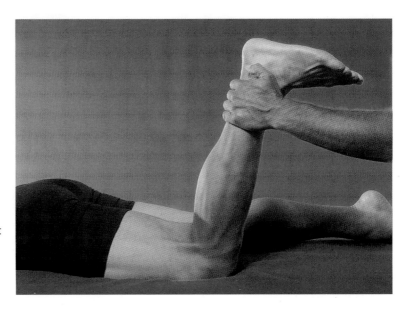

Figure 4.6 Test for hamstring muscle strain. To isolate the medial hamstring, resist knee flexion while internally rotating the leg. For isolation of the lateral hamstring, resist knee flexion while externally rotating the leg.

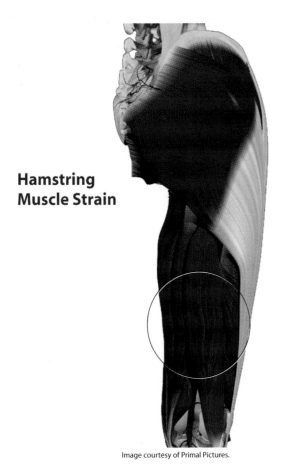

Hamstring Muscle Strain

Image courtesy of Primal Pictures.

Thigh Strain Taping

Support the quadriceps and hamstring muscles with an elastic wrap (figure 4.7) and, if necessary, supplement the wrap with elastic tape (figure 4.8). Use a 4- or 6-inch-wide (10.2- or 15.2-centimeter-wide) elastic wrap to encircle the thigh. Cover the muscle both distal and proximal to the point of strain to provide optimal support. For a high strain, you may need to incorporate a hip spica to support the proximal muscle attachment. You can also use a taping procedure alone or in combination with an elastic wrap to support a thigh strain.

Thigh Exercises

The hamstring muscles cross the hip and the knee, acting on both joints. Therefore, supplement the stretching and strengthening exercises for hip extensors with those described for knee flexors in chapter 3. Similarly, because the rectus femoris of the quadriceps group crosses both the knee and hip, include the exercises for knee extensors and hip flexors in the athlete's regimen.

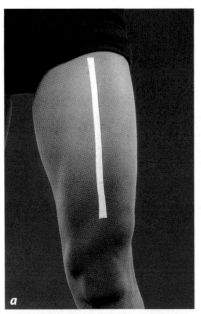
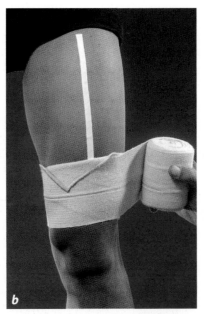
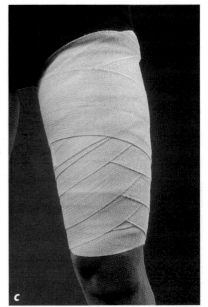

Figure 4.7   Elastic wrap to support a strain of the quadriceps muscles. *(a)* To prevent slipping of the wrap, apply tape adherent, or roll tape into a small strip and apply the roll to the thigh before applying the wrap. *(b-c)* Apply the wrap in a circular pattern around the thigh. Adhesive tape may also be used to provide support to a strained thigh, which is then encircled with an elastic wrap.   *(continued)*

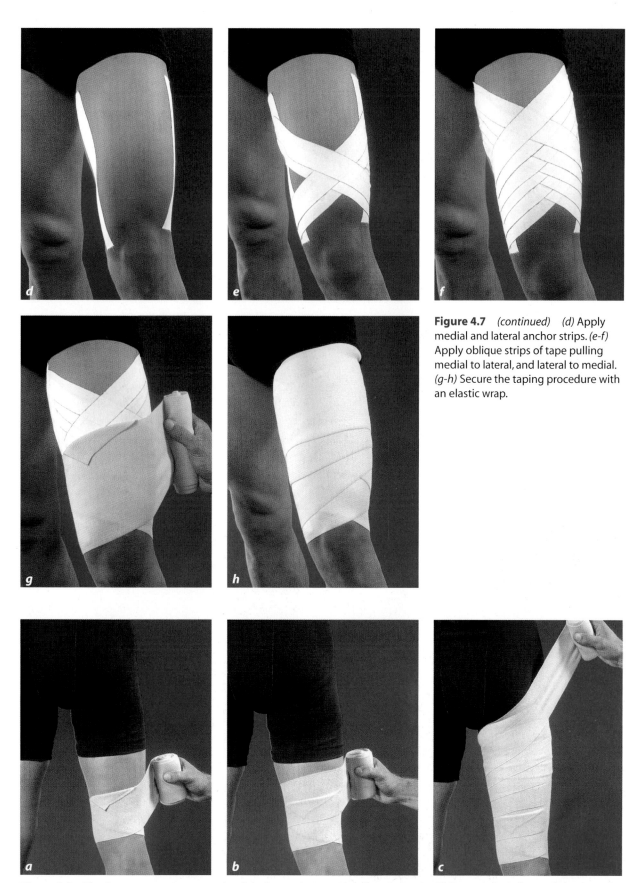

Figure 4.7 *(continued) (d)* Apply medial and lateral anchor strips. *(e-f)* Apply oblique strips of tape pulling medial to lateral, and lateral to medial. *(g-h)* Secure the taping procedure with an elastic wrap.

Figure 4.8 Elastic wrap to support a strain of the hamstring muscles. First, determine if the strain is to the medial or lateral hamstrings. If the medial hamstrings are involved, *(a)* begin by pulling the muscle toward the midline of the posterior thigh, and *(b)* then continue in a circular pattern from the distal to proximal thigh. *(continued)*

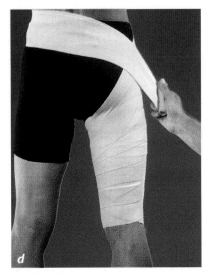
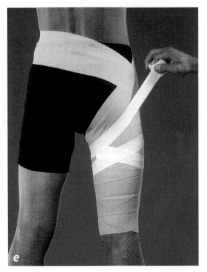
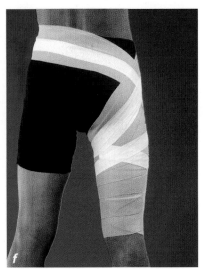

Figure 4.8 *(continued)* *(c-d)* Because the hamstring muscles attach deep beneath the buttock, the wrap will probably be more effective if applied in combination with a hip spica. *(e-f)* Trace the wrap with elastic tape.

HIP AND THIGH CONTUSIONS

Hip and thigh contusions involve the **iliac crest** (hip pointer) or quadriceps muscles of the anterior thigh. Iliac crest injuries, although painful, are not serious. Quadriceps contusions require your special attention because they can create a condition known as **myositis ossificans,** the calcification of the **hematoma** caused by a quadriceps bruise.

iliac crest—The superior border of the iliac bone; the colloquial term for a contusion to this area is hip pointer.

myositis ossificans—The formation of bone within a muscle that has suffered a contusion.

hematoma—A collection of pooling blood.

Iliac Crest Contusion (Hip Pointer)

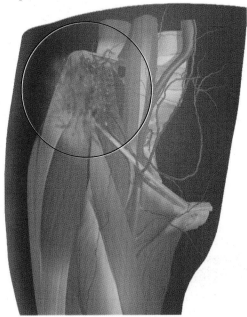

Image courtesy of Primal Pictures.

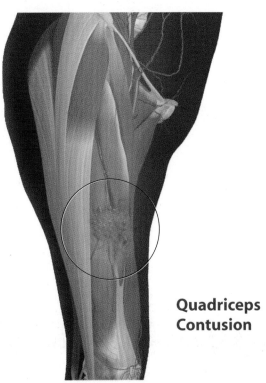

Quadriceps Contusion

Image courtesy of Primal Pictures.

Hip and Thigh Padding

Use elastic wraps and tape to secure protective pads over the iliac crest or anterior thigh. Figure 4.9 illustrates two ways to position a protective pad over the iliac crest—first with an elastic wrap and then with an elastic wrap and tape hip spica. Figure 4.10 demonstrates how elastic wrap and tape hold a protective pad over the quadriceps.

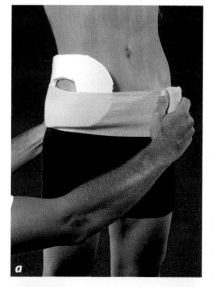

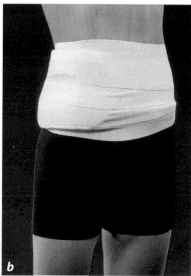

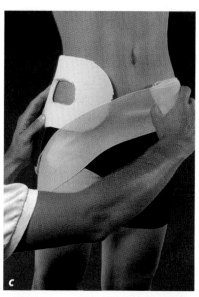

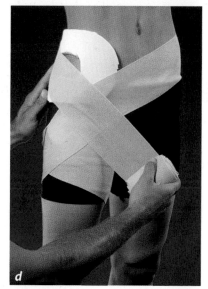

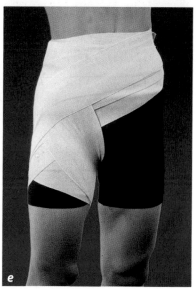

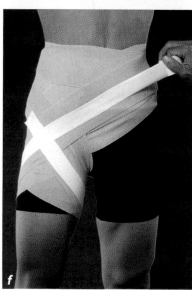

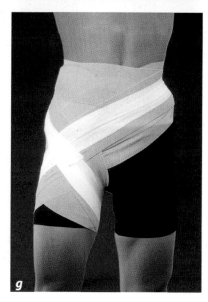

Figure 4.9 An elastic wrap to secure a protective pad over the iliac crest. *(a-b)* Position a pad over the contused iliac crest (hip pointer) and hold it in place with an elastic wrap. *(c-e)* Use a hip spica to provide additional support to the area and to hold the pad in position. *(f-g)* Trace the wrap with elastic tape.

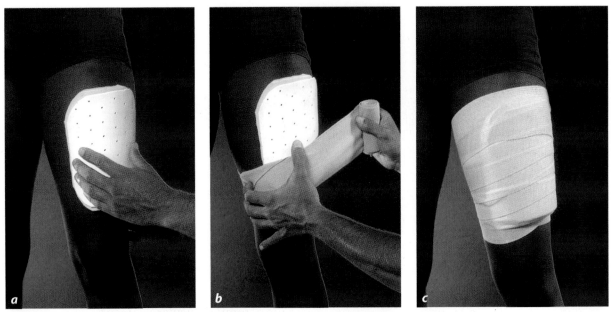

Figure 4.10 *(a-c)* An elastic wrap to secure a protective pad over the quadriceps muscles.

Hip and Thigh Contusion Exercises

The athlete should exercise to maintain normal strength and range of motion while hip and thigh contusions heal. Prescribe the stretching and strengthening exercises for both the quadriceps (chapter 3) and hip. Experienced clinicians should monitor serious thigh contusions for the onset of myositis ossificans.

CHAPTER 5

The Shoulder and Arm

The bones of the shoulder girdle include the clavicle, scapula, and humerus. The proximal clavicle and sternum form the sternoclavicular joint, which is the only articulation of the upper extremity with the trunk. The anterior and posterior sternoclavicular, the costoclavicular, and the interclavicular ligaments stabilize the joint. The distal clavicle and the acromion process of the scapula create the acromioclavicular joint, an

articulation reinforced by the coracoclavicular and acromioclavicular ligaments.

The glenoid cavity of the scapula and the head of the humerus form the shoulder, also known as the glenohumeral joint. The glenoid labrum, the glenohumeral ligaments, and the joint capsule reinforce this shallow, unstable ball-and-socket articulation.

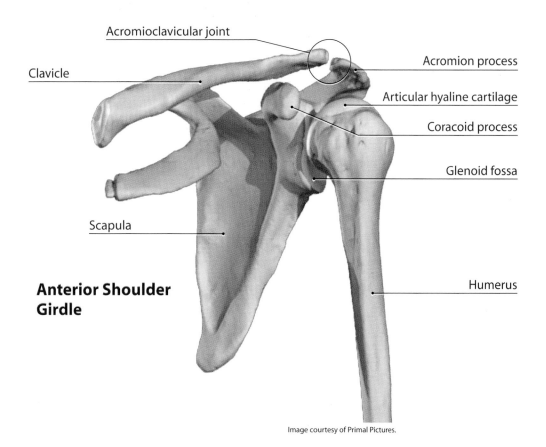

Acromioclavicular joint

Clavicle

Acromion process

Articular hyaline cartilage

Coracoid process

Glenoid fossa

Scapula

Anterior Shoulder Girdle

Humerus

Image courtesy of Primal Pictures.

Posterior Shoulder Girdle

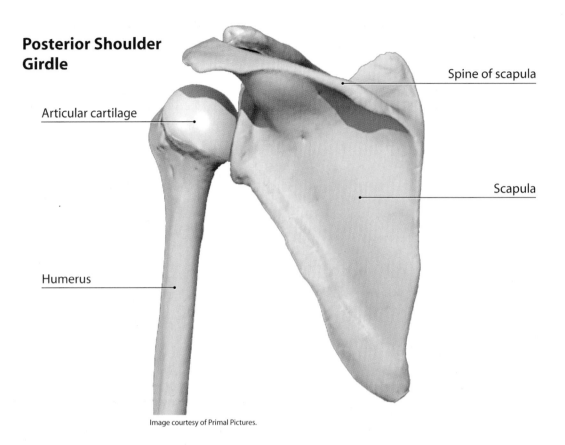

Articular cartilage

Spine of scapula

Scapula

Humerus

Image courtesy of Primal Pictures.

Shoulder Complex Ligaments

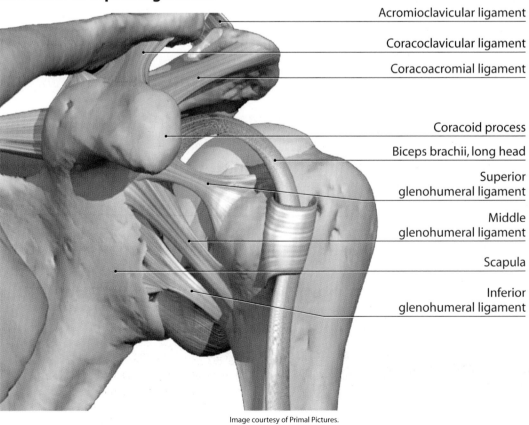

Acromioclavicular ligament

Coracoclavicular ligament

Coracoacromial ligament

Coracoid process

Biceps brachii, long head

Superior
glenohumeral ligament

Middle
glenohumeral ligament

Scapula

Inferior
glenohumeral ligament

Image courtesy of Primal Pictures.

The pectoralis major (clavicular portion) and the anterior deltoid produce flexion. Extension results from the latissimus dorsi, teres major, and pectoralis major (sternal portion). Abduction occurs with the deltoid and the **rotator cuff**, whose muscles include the subscapularis, supraspinatus, infraspinatus, and teres minor (figure 5.1).

> **rotator cuff**—The muscle group in the shoulder consisting of the subscapularis, supraspinatus, infraspinatus, and teres minor.

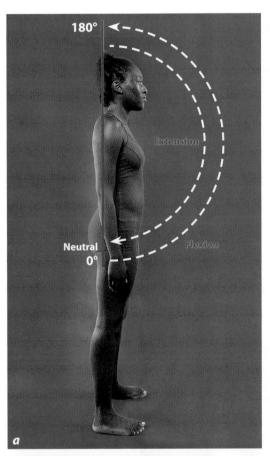

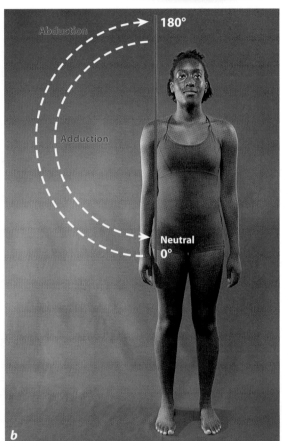

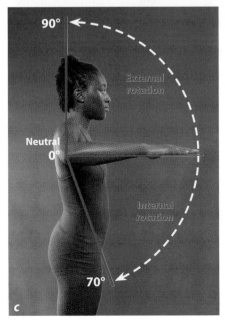

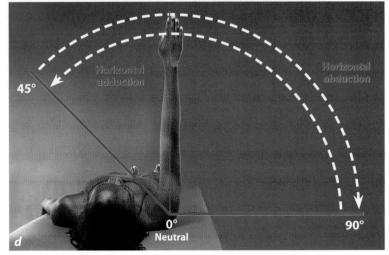

Figure 5.1 *(a)* Shoulder (glenohumeral) flexion and extension ranges of motion; *(b)* shoulder abduction and adduction ranges of motion; *(c)* shoulder internal and external rotation ranges of motion; *(d)* shoulder horizontal adduction and abduction ranges of motion. *(continued)*

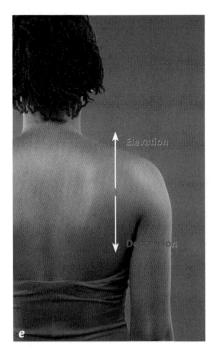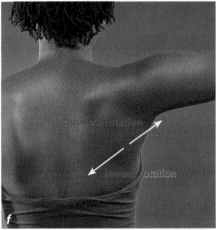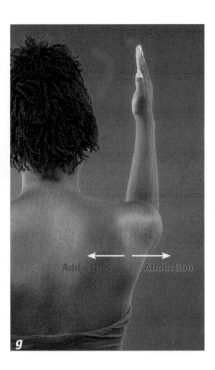

Figure 5.1 *(continued)* Scapular ranges of motion include *(e)* scapular elevation and depression *(f)* outward and inward rotation; *(g)* abduction and adduction.

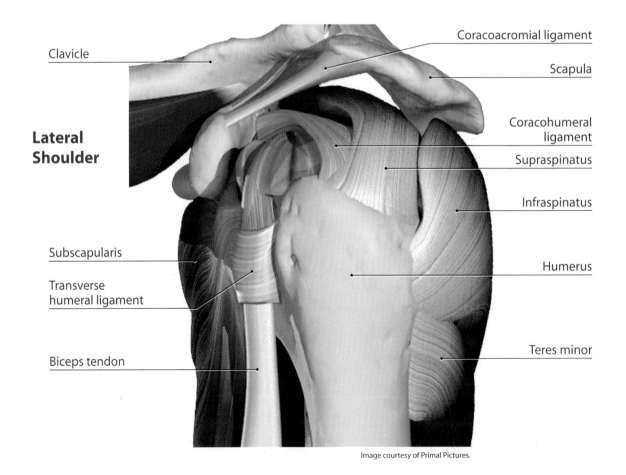

Lateral Shoulder

Clavicle

Coracoacromial ligament

Scapula

Coracohumeral ligament

Supraspinatus

Infraspinatus

Subscapularis

Transverse humeral ligament

Humerus

Biceps tendon

Teres minor

Image courtesy of Primal Pictures.

The contraction of the pectoralis major (sternal portion), latissimus dorsi, and teres major muscles causes adduction. The action of the subscapularis and pectoralis major muscles precipitates internal rotation, and the SIT muscles of the rotator cuff—the supraspinatus, infraspinatus, and teres minor—induce external rotation.

Horizontal flexion occurs with the combination of the coracobrachialis, pectoralis major, and deltoid (anterior portion), and horizontal extension depends on the infraspinatus, teres minor, and deltoid (posterior portion).

The movement of the glenohumeral joint occurs in conjunction with the movement of the scapula. The range of the scapula includes abduction (pectoralis minor and serratus anterior muscles) and adduction (rhomboid muscles), outward rotation (serratus anterior and trapezius muscles) and inward rotation (pectoralis minor and rhomboid muscles), as well as elevation (levator scapulae) and depression (pectoralis minor muscle).

Key Palpation Landmarks

Anterior
- ▸ Deltoid muscle
- ▸ Pectoralis major muscle
- ▸ Clavicle

Posterior
- ▸ Scapula

Superior
- ▸ Acromioclavicular joint

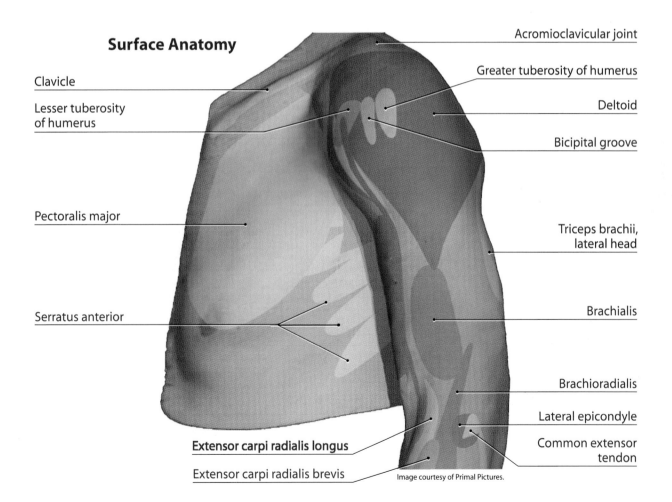

Surface Anatomy

Clavicle

Lesser tuberosity of humerus

Pectoralis major

Serratus anterior

Extensor carpi radialis longus

Extensor carpi radialis brevis

Acromioclavicular joint

Greater tuberosity of humerus

Deltoid

Bicipital groove

Triceps brachii, lateral head

Brachialis

Brachioradialis

Lateral epicondyle

Common extensor tendon

Image courtesy of Primal Pictures.

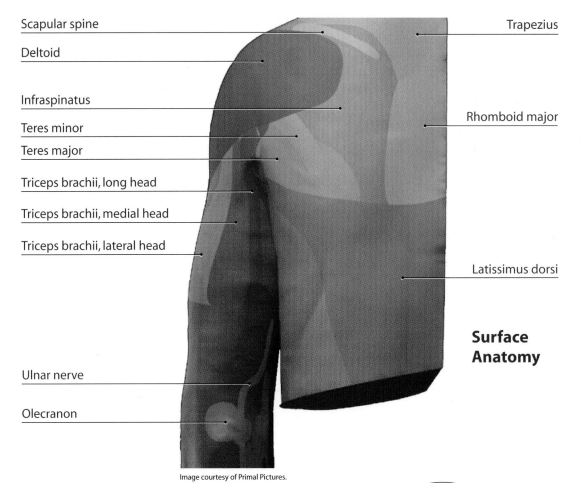

Scapular spine

Deltoid

Infraspinatus

Teres minor

Teres major

Triceps brachii, long head

Triceps brachii, medial head

Triceps brachii, lateral head

Ulnar nerve

Olecranon

Trapezius

Rhomboid major

Latissimus dorsi

Surface Anatomy

Image courtesy of Primal Pictures.

ACROMIOCLAVICULAR JOINT SPRAINS

Athletes suffer an **acromioclavicular joint sprain** (known colloquially as a separated shoulder) when they fall on the hand, elbow, or the shoulder itself. Clinicians categorize the sprains as first- to third-degree injuries. The first degree describes a minor tear of the acromioclavicular ligament, and the third degree refers to a complete rupture of both the acromioclavicular and coracoclavicular ligaments. In the latter case, the shoulder drops and the clavicle protrudes against the skin of the superior shoulder.

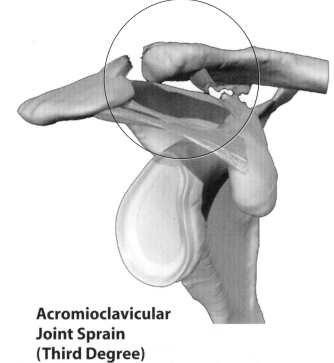

Acromioclavicular Joint Sprain (Third Degree)

Acromioclavicular Joint Taping

Begin taping an acromioclavicular joint sprain by placing anchor strips around the arm, over the top of the shoulder, and on the chest and back (figure 5.2). Make certain that when taping the shoulder or chest you protect the nipple with gauze or a bandage. Continue taping with successive strips from the arm anchor to the shoulder anchor and from the chest anchor to the back anchor.

acromioclavicular joint sprain—A sprain to the acromioclavicular or coracoclavicular ligaments of the joint formed by the distal clavicle and the acromion process of the scapula; also known colloquially as a separated shoulder.

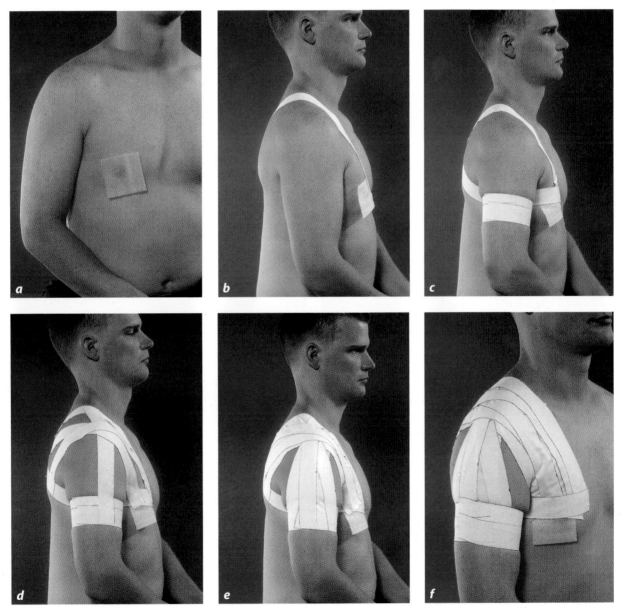

Figure 5.2 Acromioclavicular joint sprain (separated shoulder) taping. *(a)* Any taping of the shoulder or chest that has the potential to cover the nipple should begin with the application of protective dressing. *(b)* Apply anchor strips to the superior, anterior, and posterior aspects of the shoulder as well as *(c)* to the proximal arm. *(d-f)* Apply strips from the arm anchor to the superior shoulder anchor and from the anterior to posterior anchors in an overlapping fashion so that the crossing point of the tape is over the acromioclavicular joint.

You may supplement or replace this procedure by using a protective pad over the injured acromioclavicular joint. Figure 5.3 illustrates the technique for making a protective pad from orthoplast and how to secure the pad with a shoulder spica with an elastic wrap. You can use this technique for making a custom-fitted protective pad to protect other injuries, such as contusions of the quadriceps, iliac crest, and a blocker's exostosis.

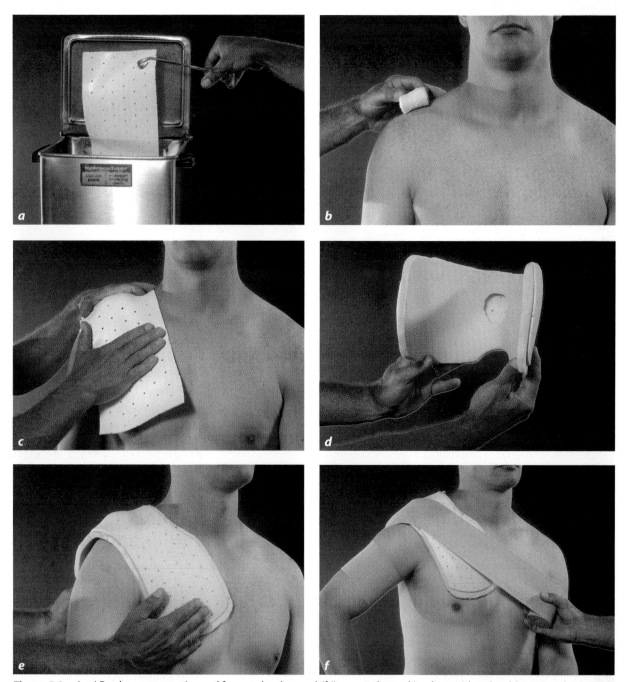

Figure 5.3 *(a-e)* Produce a protective pad from orthoplast and *(f-i)* secure the pad in place with a shoulder spica elastic wrap.

(continued)

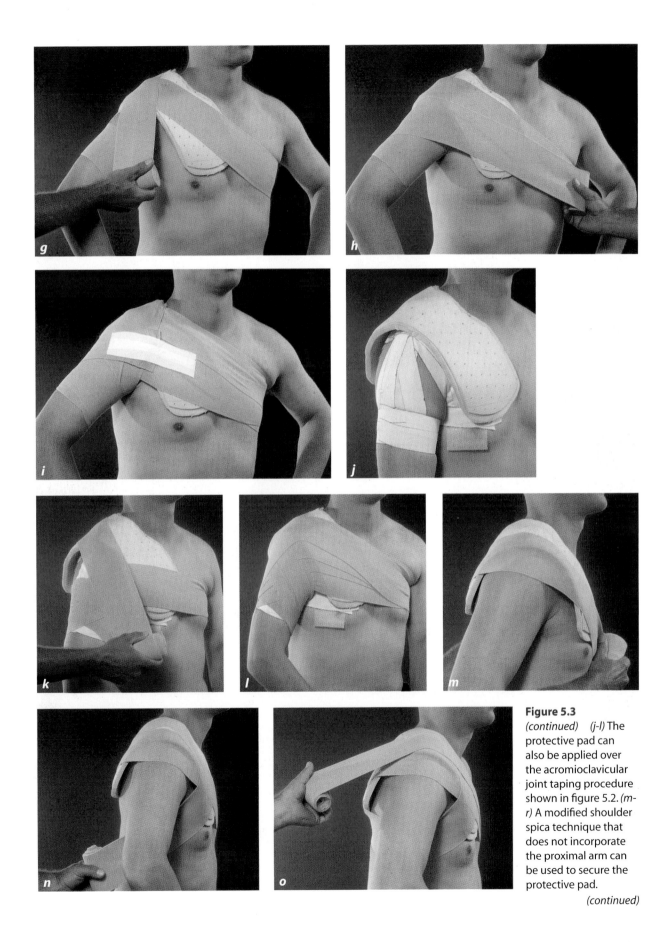

Figure 5.3
(continued) *(j-l)* The protective pad can also be applied over the acromioclavicular joint taping procedure shown in figure 5.2. *(m-r)* A modified shoulder spica technique that does not incorporate the proximal arm can be used to secure the protective pad.

(continued)

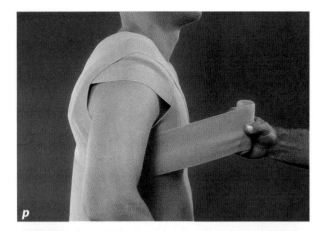

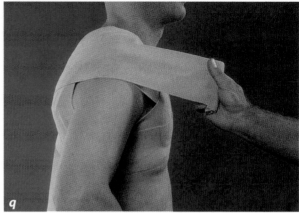

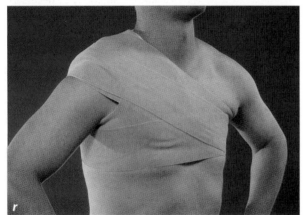

Figure 5.3   *(continued)*

McConnel Taping for Acromioclavicular Joint Sprains

You can use the same kind of tape used for McConnel taping of the patella for acromioclavicular joint sprains. This taping procedure can be left in place for an extended period and will help "reapproximate" the acromioclavicular joint (figure 5.4).

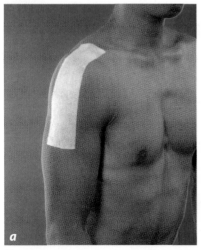
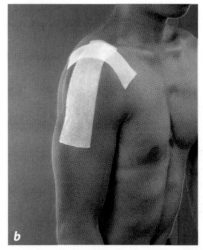
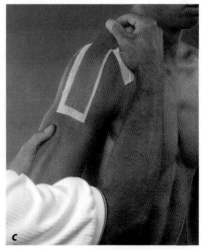

Figure 5.4   McConnel taping for an acromioclavicular joint sprain. Use Cover-Roll stretch and Leukotape as with the McConnel taping for patellofemoral joint pain. *(a)* Apply the first Cover-Roll strip vertically from the deltoid tuberosity past the acromioclavicular joint by 3/4 to 1 1/4 inches (2 to 3 centimeters). *(b)* Apply the second strip from the coracoid process to the spine of the scapula. *(c)* Apply the first Leukotape strip vertically over the Cover-Roll strip while approximating the acromioclavicular joint.   *(continued)*

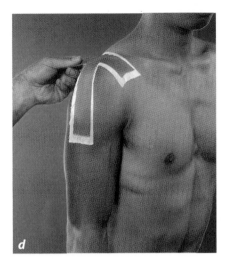

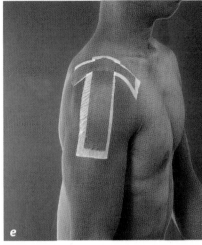

Figure 5.4 *(continued)* *(d)* Apply the second strip of Leukotape anterior to posterior. *(e)* The point of the crossing strips should center over the acromioclavicular joint. An additional layer of Leukotape strips may be necessary to provide ample support.

Shoulder Exercises

Most sports, especially those that require overhead arm motion, rely on adequate strength and flexibility of the shoulder. Construct a simple T-bar for exercises to stretch the shoulder (figure 5.5). Be certain that the exercise regimen addresses the full range of motion of the shoulder.

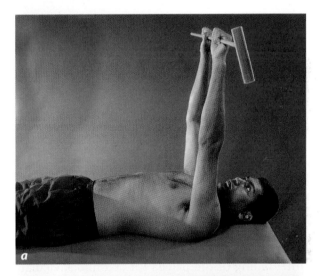

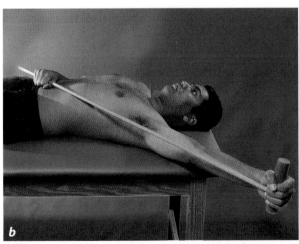

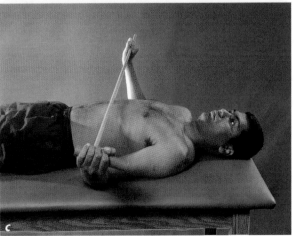

Figure 5.5 A simple T-bar to stretch the shoulder muscles through *(a)* flexion, *(b)* abduction, and *(c)* external rotation.

Strengthening exercises employ dumbbells, elastic bands, or a combination of both devices. Figure 5.6 illustrates how a hand-held weight provides resistance through each of the motions of the shoulder. Elastic bands can supply similar resistance while also allowing for exercise that traces functional movement patterns (figure 5.7).

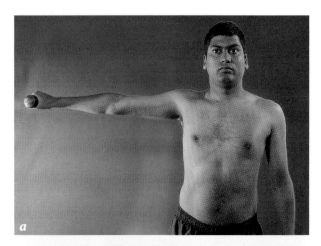

Figure 5.6   A hand-held weight to strengthen the shoulder *(a)* abductor, *(b)* flexor, and *(c)* extensor muscles. Normally, these motions should not exceed the horizontal positions seen in *(a)* and *(b)*.

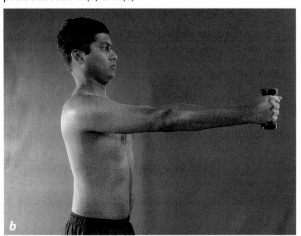

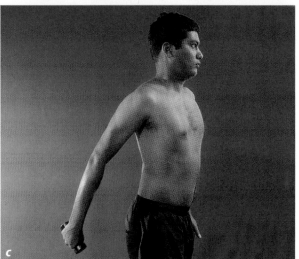

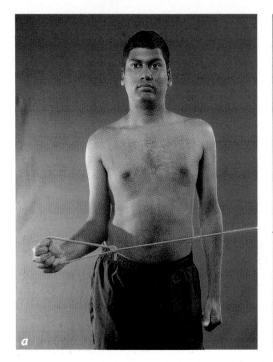

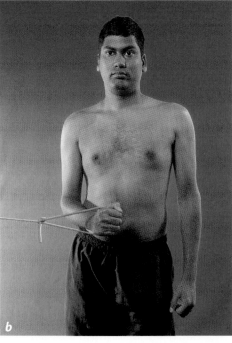

Figure 5.7   Elastic bands are effective for strengthening the shoulder *(a)* external and *(b)* internal rotator muscles.

GLENOHUMERAL SPRAINS

Sprains, **subluxations**, and **dislocations**, all common injuries of the glenohumeral joint, cause the shoulder to be chronically unstable. The athlete often requires surgery to repair the damage. Although congenital factors may contribute to the injuries, sprains or dislocations usually occur when the athlete applies an external force to the arm. Shoulder abduction and external rotation are the common mechanisms of injury for anterior dislocation.

> **subluxation**—A partial dislocation of a joint.
>
> **dislocation**—A complete separation of two articulating bones.

Shoulder Sprain or Instability Taping

Your taping procedure should prevent excessive abduction and external rotation. An elastic-wrap shoulder spica, traced with elastic tape, limits these motions (figure 5.8). Have the athlete internally rotate the shoulder and begin taping by encircling the arm and crossing over the anterior chest; this action pulls the shoulder into internal rotation and limits external rotation. The amount of mobility that the athlete requires will dictate the degree of limitation that you provide.

Shoulder braces restrict abduction and external rotation (figure 5.9). You can adjust their restriction from a light to a substantial degree.

Shoulder Sprain or Instability Exercises

Combine the exercises illustrated in figures 5.5 through 5.7 with the shoulder wrapping and bracing procedures. Do not, however, prescribe the stretching exercises that enhance shoulder abduction and external rotation, because, in this case, the exercises would stress an unstable shoulder that is already hypermobile. Have the athlete focus on internal-rotation strengthening exercises because they will limit the external rotation of the shoulder.

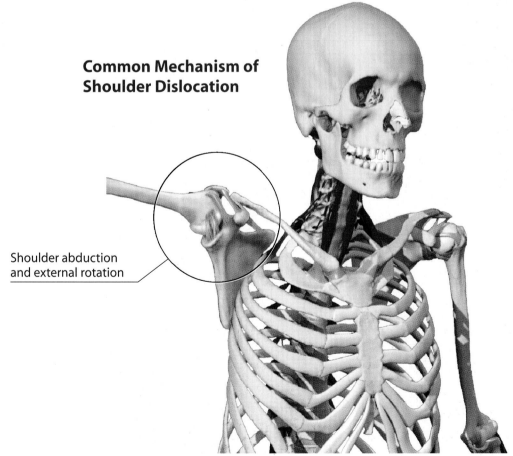

Common Mechanism of Shoulder Dislocation

Shoulder abduction and external rotation

Image courtesy of Primal Pictures.

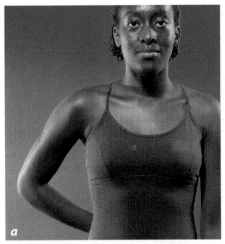

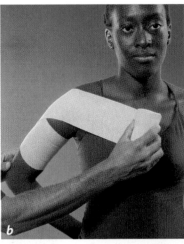

Figure 5.8 A shoulder spica with elastic wrap and tape to support the unstable shoulder. *(a)* The procedure begins by having the athlete place the shoulder in an internally rotated position with the hand on the hip. *(b)* Start the wrap on the arm and pull medially across the anterior chest. *(c-e)* The wrap continues around the arm and again proceeds around the chest. *(f-h)* Use elastic tape to trace the elastic wrap.

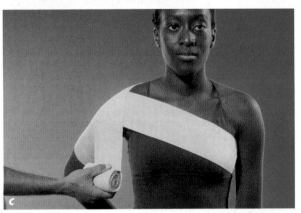

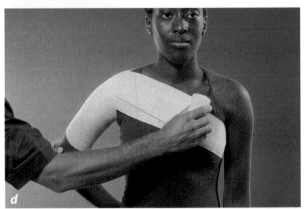

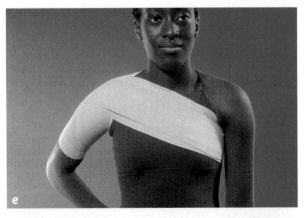

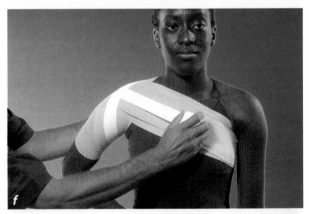

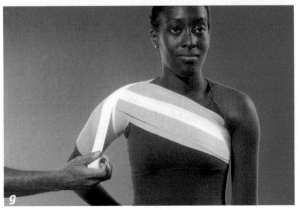

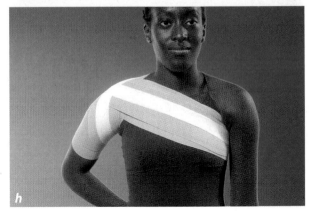

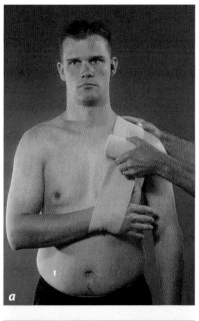

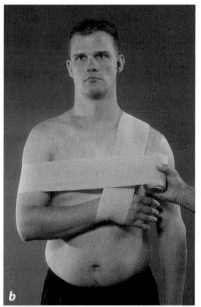

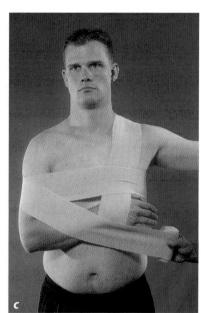

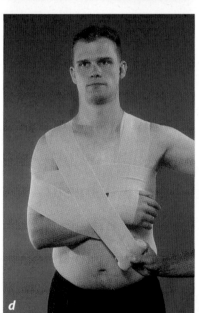

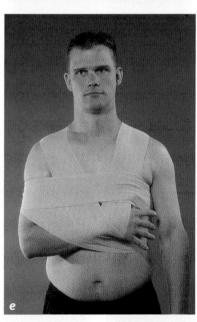

Figure 5.9 *(a-e)* An elastic wrap can immobilize an acutely injured shoulder. *(f-g)* A commercially produced brace can limit shoulder abduction and external rotation. Control the degree of abduction through the adjustable straps of the brace.

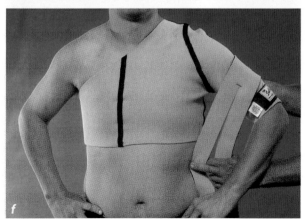

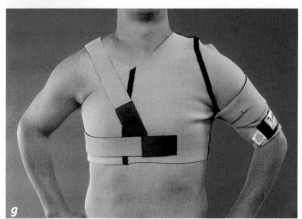

ARM CONTUSIONS

Athletes often suffer arm contusions, especially when playing football or other contact sports. Arm contusions, like those of the thigh, may develop myositis ossificans, an injury termed blocker's **exostosis.**

exostosis—Abnormal bone growth.

Arm Contusion Taping

Protect the arm from repeated trauma by securing a protective pad to the area. Figure 5.10 illustrates how to use elastic tape when applying a protective pad to the lateral aspect of the arm.

Arm Contusion Exercises

The exercises illustrated in figures 5.5 through 5.7 and those for the elbow in chapter 6 will help the injured athlete maintain normal strength and flexibility. An experienced clinician should monitor the injury for exostosis in the soft tissue of the arm and prescribe rest if this condition develops.

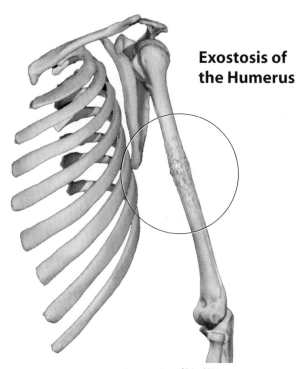

Exostosis of the Humerus

Image courtesy of Primal Pictures.

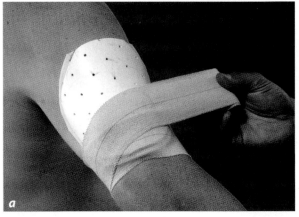 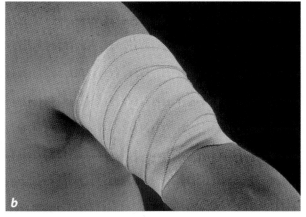

Figure 5.10 *(a-b)* Elastic tape to secure a protective pad to the arm.

CHAPTER 6

The Elbow and Forearm

T he joining of the distal humerus with the proximal ulna forms the elbow. The medial collateral ligament, called the ulnar, and lateral collateral ligament, referred to as the radial, limit valgus and varus displacement, respectively.

Anterior Elbow

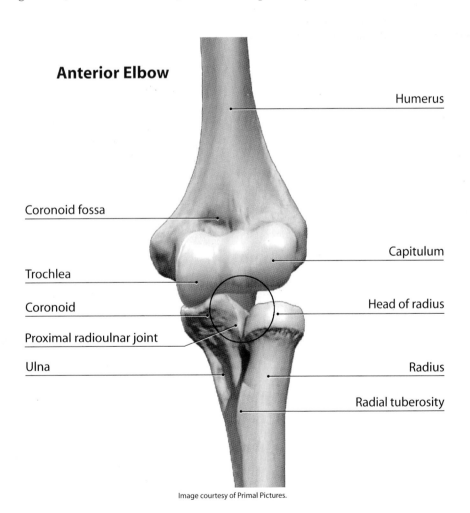

Humerus

Coronoid fossa

Capitulum

Trochlea

Coronoid

Head of radius

Proximal radioulnar joint

Ulna

Radius

Radial tuberosity

Image courtesy of Primal Pictures.

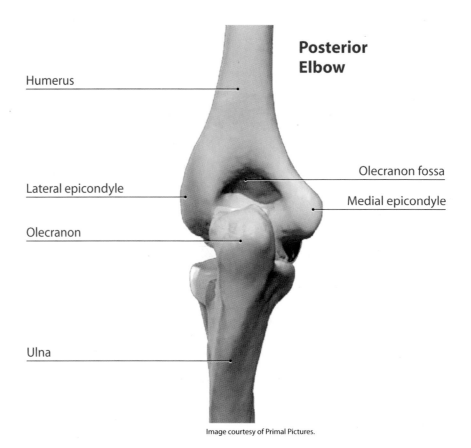

Posterior Elbow

Humerus

Lateral epicondyle

Olecranon

Ulna

Olecranon fossa

Medial epicondyle

Image courtesy of Primal Pictures.

Elbow Joint Ligaments

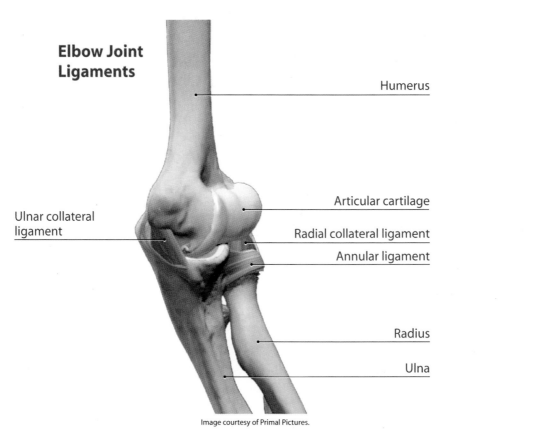

Humerus

Ulnar collateral ligament

Articular cartilage

Radial collateral ligament

Annular ligament

Radius

Ulna

Image courtesy of Primal Pictures.

The hinge of the elbow permits flexion and extension (figure 6.1). Flexion occurs through the action of the anterior muscles of the arm, which include the biceps brachii and brachialis. The three heads of the triceps brachii comprise the posterior muscles and produce elbow extension.

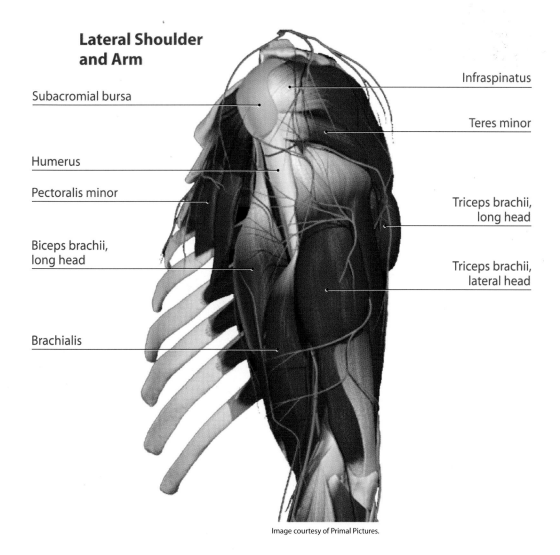

Lateral Shoulder and Arm

Subacromial bursa

Humerus

Pectoralis minor

Biceps brachii, long head

Brachialis

Infraspinatus

Teres minor

Triceps brachii, long head

Triceps brachii, lateral head

Image courtesy of Primal Pictures.

The radius and ulna of the forearm create three joints: the proximal radioulnar, the distal radioulnar, and the articulation along the shafts of both bones. The fibers of the annular ligament stabilize the proximal radioulnar joint. The interosseous membrane joins the shafts of the radius and ulna, and an articular capsule supports the distal radioulnar joint. Pronation and supination describe the potential movements of the forearm (figure 6.1). The pronator teres and pronator quadratus muscles cause pronation, and the supinator muscle produces supination.

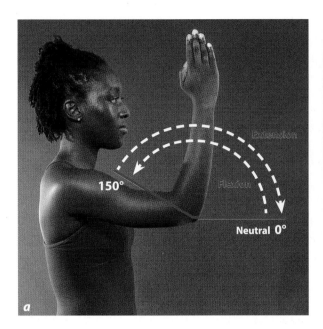

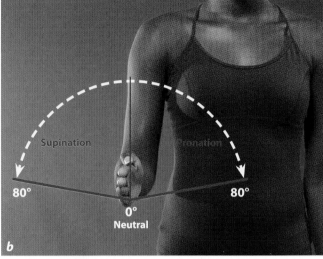

Figure 6.1 *(a)* Elbow flexion and extension ranges of motion; *(b)* forearm pronation and supination ranges of motion.

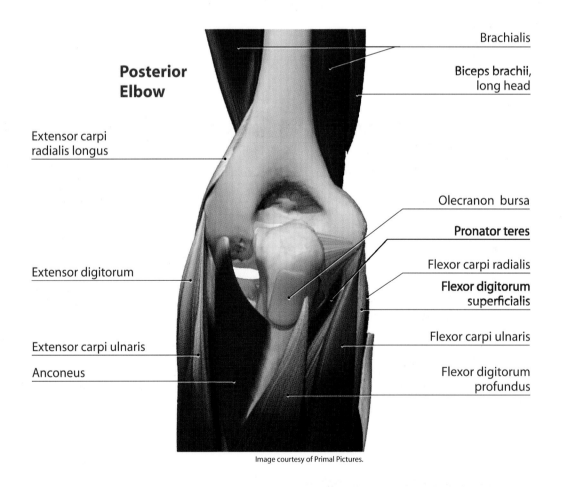

Posterior Elbow

Brachialis

Biceps brachii, long head

Extensor carpi radialis longus

Olecranon bursa

Pronator teres

Extensor digitorum

Flexor carpi radialis

Flexor digitorum superficialis

Flexor carpi ulnaris

Extensor carpi ulnaris

Anconeus

Flexor digitorum profundus

Image courtesy of Primal Pictures.

Key Palpation Landmarks

Anterior
▸ Cubital fossa
▸ Biceps tendon

Medial
▸ Ulnar nerve
▸ Wrist flexor-pronator group
▸ Medial epicondyle
▸ Medial collateral ligament

Lateral
▸ Wrist extensor-supinator muscle group
▸ Lateral epicondyle
▸ Lateral collateral ligament

Posterior
▸ Olecranon process
▸ Olecranon bursa
▸ Triceps muscle

ELBOW SPRAINS

Similar to knee injuries, elbow sprains occur when valgus or varus forces damage the medial or lateral collateral ligaments, respectively. Sports that depend on the athlete's overarm throwing ability will impart chronic stress to the medial compartment of the elbow and injure the medial collateral ligament.

Elbow Sprain Taping

Medial and lateral instabilities can be difficult injuries to support, and taping the elbow is unlikely to help the athlete who suffers from chronic stress to the medial collateral ligament. Figure 6.2, however, illustrates a collateral ligament taping procedure that you may find valuable for some cases. The procedure is remarkably similar to taping the collateral ligaments of the knee (chapter 3).

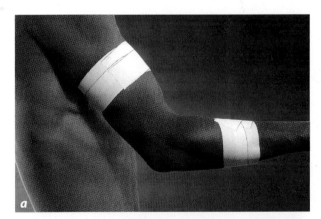

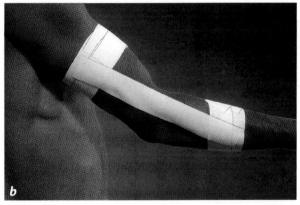

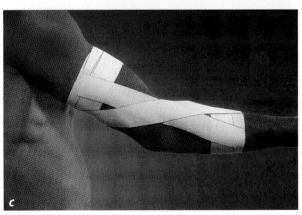

Figure 6.2 Elbow collateral ligament taping for instability of the lateral collateral ligament. *(a)* The procedure begins with proximal and distal anchor strips. *(b-d)* Place strips over the lateral collateral ligament in an X fashion. *(continued)*

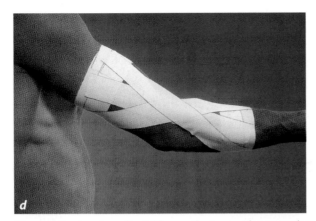
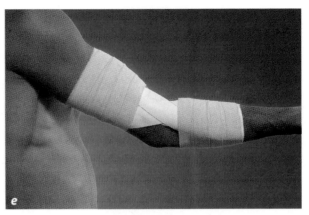

Figure 6.2   *(continued)*   *(e)* Secure the tape with proximal and distal anchors using elastic tape that encloses all but the elbow joint itself.

Elbow Exercises

Stretch the elbow flexor and extensor muscles with the assistance of the contralateral extremity (figure 6.3).

Strengthening exercises should work the muscles that produce elbow flexion and extension, forearm pronation and supination, and wrist flexion and extension. I recommend a combination of hand-held weights and elastic bands, as figure 6.4 illustrates. Chapter 7 will discuss exercises for the wrist.

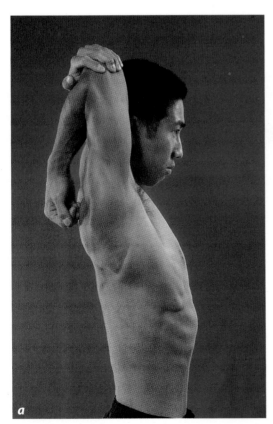
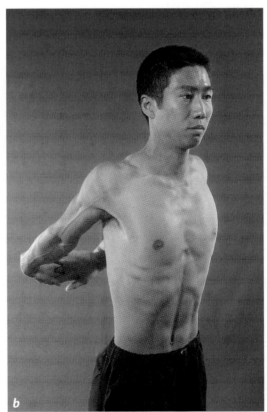

Figure 6.3   Stretching of the elbow *(a)* extensor and *(b)* flexor muscles with the contralateral extremity.

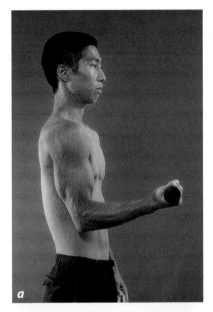

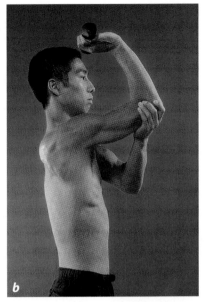

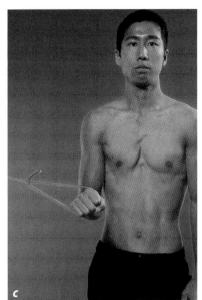

Figure 6.4 Strengthening exercises for the elbow *(a)* flexor and *(b)* extensor muscles with a hand-held weight. Elastic bands will strengthen the forearm *(c)* pronator and *(d)* supinator muscles.

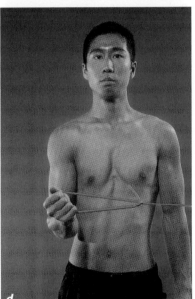

Elbow Hyperextension Injury

ELBOW HYPEREXTENSION

Self-inflicted or external forces can extend the elbow beyond its normal anatomical limit; the motion produces a hyperextension injury that damages the ulna or humerus where it articulates during extension. The soft-tissue structures on the anterior aspect of the elbow could also suffer trauma. In severe cases, hyperextension will fracture or dislocate the elbow.

Elbow Hyperextension Taping

Elbow and knee hyperextension share a similar taping procedure (chapter 3). Determine the degree of extension that produces discomfort and slightly flex the joint for the duration of the taping. Place anchor strips around the arm and forearm (figure 6.5). To prevent slippage, I recommend that you apply the anchors directly to the skin. You may also find it advantageous to secure the proximal anchor above the belly of the biceps. Tape successive, interlocking strips over the anterior aspect of the elbow. Elastic tape works well when supporting hyperextension injuries. If necessary, complete the taping procedure by enclosing the elbow with elastic tape or wrap.

Hyperextension Exercises

Figure 6.3 details extension and flexion exercises that will restore the normal range of motion of the injured elbow. The strengthening regimen needs to isolate the elbow flexor and extensor muscles (see figure 6.4).

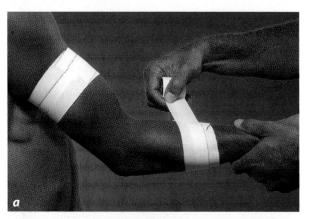

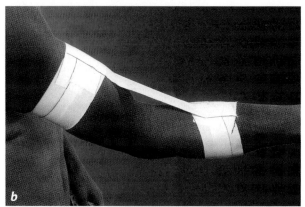

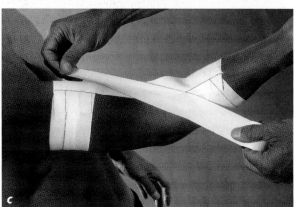

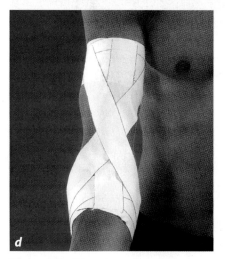

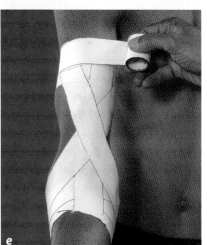

Figure 6.5　Elbow hyperextension taping procedure. *(a)* Begin the procedure on a shaved arm and apply proximal and distal anchor strips. *(b-d)* Form an X with three strips of tape over the anterior aspect of the elbow. *(e)* Apply proximal and distal anchor strips to secure the tape.　*(continued)*

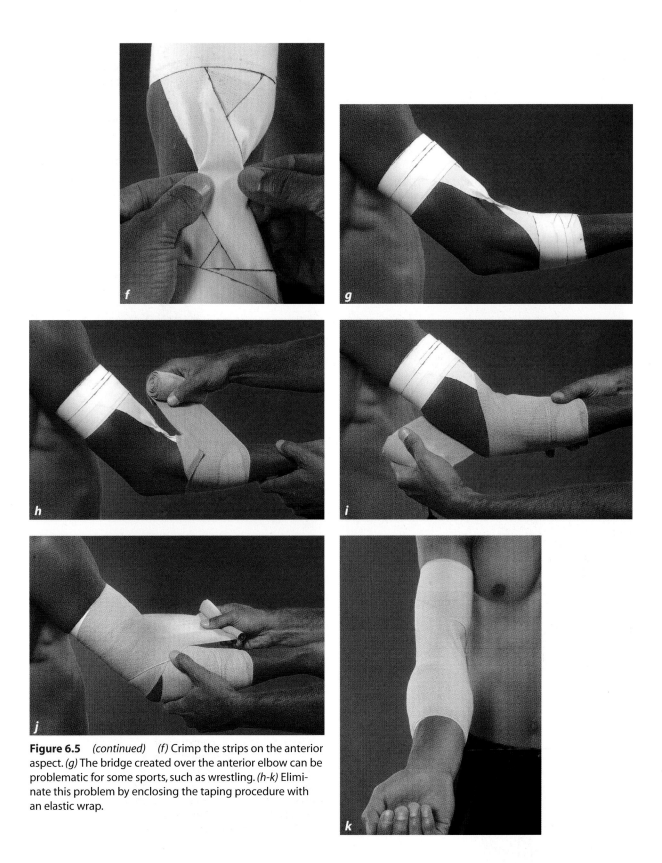

Figure 6.5 *(continued)* *(f)* Crimp the strips on the anterior aspect. *(g)* The bridge created over the anterior elbow can be problematic for some sports, such as wrestling. *(h-k)* Eliminate this problem by enclosing the taping procedure with an elastic wrap.

EPICONDYLITIS OF THE HUMERUS

The medial and lateral epicondyles of the humerus attach several muscles. Muscles originate from the lateral epicondyle for forearm supination and wrist extension. The medial epicondyle joins muscles for forearm pronation and wrist flexion. Repetitive forearm and wrist motion—such as that required for tennis or throwing—inflames these muscles at their points of origin from the medial or lateral epicondyles. Tennis players commonly suffer from lateral **epicondylitis**, known colloquially as tennis elbow. Athletes who repeatedly use a throwing motion, especially adolescents, frequently experience medial epicondylitis, often called Little Leaguer's elbow.

Epicondylitis Taping

I have found that taping for epicondylitis is not always effective. Some patients experience relief from strips of tape applied to compress the proximal forearm (figure 6.6). Commercially produced straps will also serve this purpose (figure 6.7).

Exercise caution when treating the adolescent patient with medial epicondylitis. For many adolescents, the strength of the muscles exceeds the tolerance of the immature bone. The throwing mechanism may cause **avulsion** fractures of the medial epicondyle. For this reason, do not tape

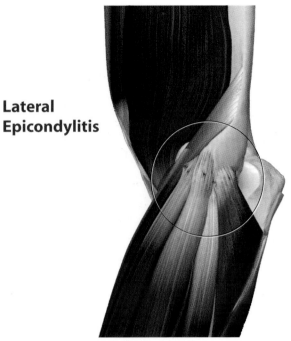

Lateral Epicondylitis

Image courtesy of Primal Pictures.

an adolescent athlete so that he or she throws through the discomfort associated with medial epicondylitis.

epicondylitis—Inflammation of an epicondyle.

avulsion—The tearing away of a tendon or ligament attachment from bone.

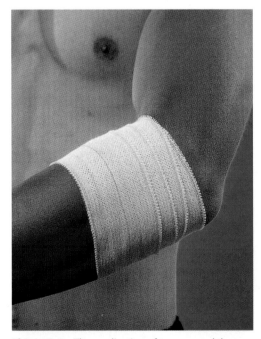

Figure 6.6   The application of tape around the proximal forearm can sometimes alleviate pain associated with lateral epicondylitis (tennis elbow).

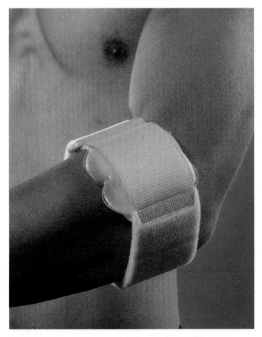

Figure 6.7   A commercially produced brace can also alleviate pain associated with lateral epicondylitis.

Epicondylitis Exercises

After the inflammation associated with lateral epicondylitis has resolved, prescribe exercises to enhance the athlete's range of motion and strength. The stretching exercises for the elbow and forearm will increase flexibility. For lateral epicondylitis, hyperflex the wrist during complete pronation (figure 6.8). The strengthening techniques should exercise the forearm supinators and wrist extensors (chapter 7). Rest is the best treatment for medial epicondylitis.

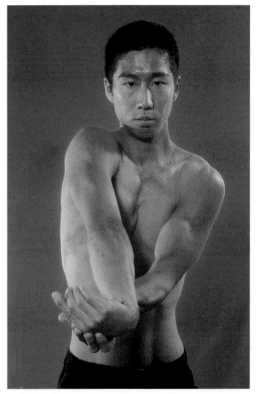

Figure 6.8 Stretching of the extensor-supinator muscles commonly implicated in lateral epicondylitis.

The Wrist and Hand

The wrist has two rows of carpal bones. The proximal row contains the scaphoid, lunate, triquetral, and pisiform bones. The trapezium, trapezoid, capitate, and hamate bones complete the distal row. The hand includes five metacar-pal bones, and the fingers have 14 phalanges: a proximal and distal phalanx in the thumb and a proximal, middle, and distal phalanx in each of the four fingers.

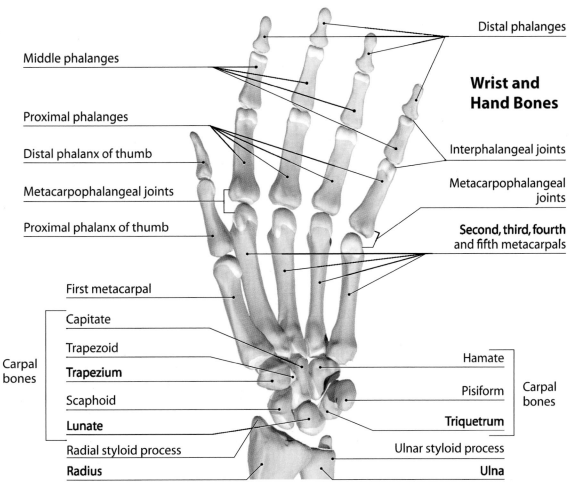

Middle phalanges

Proximal phalanges

Distal phalanx of thumb

Metacarpophalangeal joints

Proximal phalanx of thumb

First metacarpal

Carpal bones

Capitate

Trapezoid

Trapezium

Scaphoid

Lunate

Radial styloid process

Radius

Distal phalanges

Wrist and Hand Bones

Interphalangeal joints

Metacarpophalangeal joints

Second, third, fourth and fifth metacarpals

Hamate

Pisiform

Carpal bones

Triquetrum

Ulnar styloid process

Ulna

Image courtesy of Primal Pictures.

The distal radius and the scaphoid and lunate proximal carpal bones create the wrist joint, allowing movements that include flexion, extension, radial deviation (abduction), and ulnar deviation (adduction) (figure 7.1). The distal carpal bones and the metacarpals form the carpometacarpal joints. The distal ends of the metacarpals and the proximal phalanges of the fingers create the metacarpophalangeal joints. These joints flex, extend, abduct, and adduct. Each of the four fingers contain two joints: the proximal interphalangeal (PIP) and the distal interphalangeal (DIP). The interphalangeal joints permit flexion and extension. A complex network of ligaments and joint capsules supports all the joints in the hand and fingers.

The thumb is crucial because it provides specialized dexterity. The carpometacarpal joint of the thumb permits extension, flexion, abduction, adduction, opposition (figure 7.1), and reposition. The metacarpophalangeal and interphalangeal joints of the thumb permit flexion and extension.

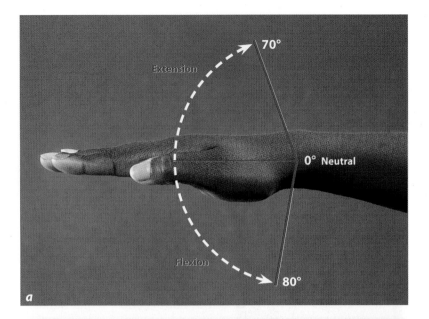

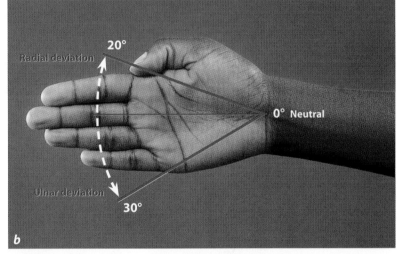

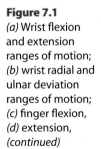**Figure 7.1**
(a) Wrist flexion and extension ranges of motion; (b) wrist radial and ulnar deviation ranges of motion; (c) finger flexion, (d) extension, (continued)

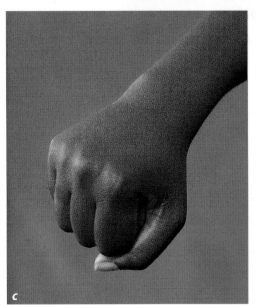

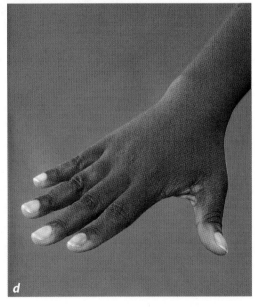

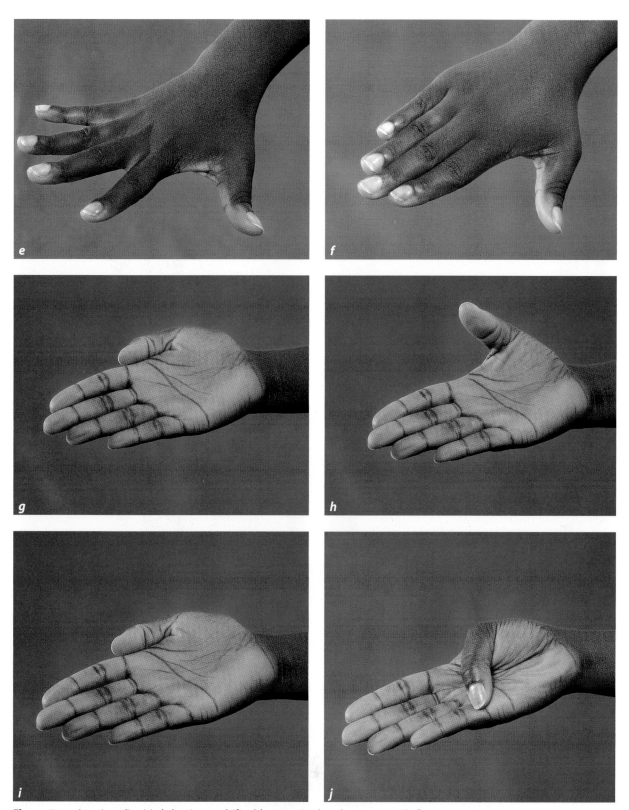

Figure 7.1 *(continued)* *(e)* abduction, and *(f)* adduction; *(g)* thumb extension, *(h)* flexion, *(i)* adduction, and *(j)* opposition.

Ligaments of the Wrist and Hand

Dorsal carpometacarpal ligaments

Lateral ligament of the trapeziometacarpal joint

Palmar intercarpal ligaments

Dorsal intercarpal ligament

Radial collateral ligament

Dorsal radiocarpal ligament

Image courtesy of Primal Pictures.

Anterior Forearm

Extensor pollicis brevis

Abductor pollicis longus

Pronator quadratus

Flexor pollicis longus

Extensor digitorum

Flexor digitorum superficialis

Extensor carpi radialis brevis

Flexor carpi radialis

Extensor carpi radialis longus

Pronator teres

Image courtesy of Primal Pictures.

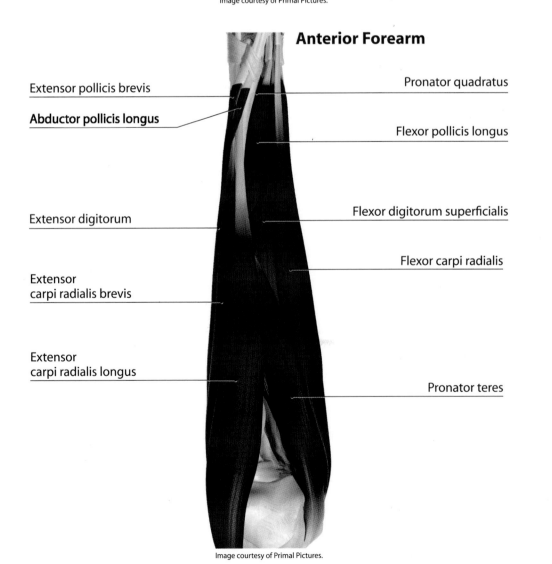

Several ligaments reinforce the joints. The ulnar collateral ligament of the metacarpophalangeal joint, which prevents valgus displacement, needs consideration with respect to athletic injury.

Several muscles originate in the forearm and hand that produce wrist, hand, and finger movement. The flexor carpi ulnaris and the flexor carpi radialis cause wrist flexion, and the contraction of the extensor carpi ulnaris and the extensor carpi radialis longus and brevis produce wrist extension. The simultaneous contraction in the wrist of the flexor carpi ulnaris and the extensor carpi ulnaris results in ulnar deviation. Conversely, if the flexor carpi radialis and the extensor carpi radialis longus contract together, radial deviation occurs. Several muscles that act on the wrist begin from the humerus and cross the elbow joint. They are, therefore, significant for normal function of both the elbow and the forearm.

Three muscles produce movement in the four fingers (figure 7.1). The flexor digitorum profundus and superficialis cause flexion; the extensor digitorum precipitates extension. The flexor digitorum profundus attaches to the distal phalanx of the fingers, and the flexor digitorum superficialis **inserts** into the middle phalanx. The first muscle flexes both the PIP and DIP joints, but the latter muscle flexes only the PIP. Both muscles, however, flex all the joints of the wrist and hand as they pass to the fingers. The insertion of the extensor digitorum gives three tendinous slips to each of the four fingers. A central tendon attaches to the middle phalanx, and two lateral bands pass to the distal phalanx. Along with some of the intrinsic muscles of the hand, this mechanism creates the **extensor hood.**

insertion—The point where muscle attaches to bone; usually refers to the distal attachment of the muscle.

extensor hood—The anatomical tendon configuration on the dorsal aspect of the finger.

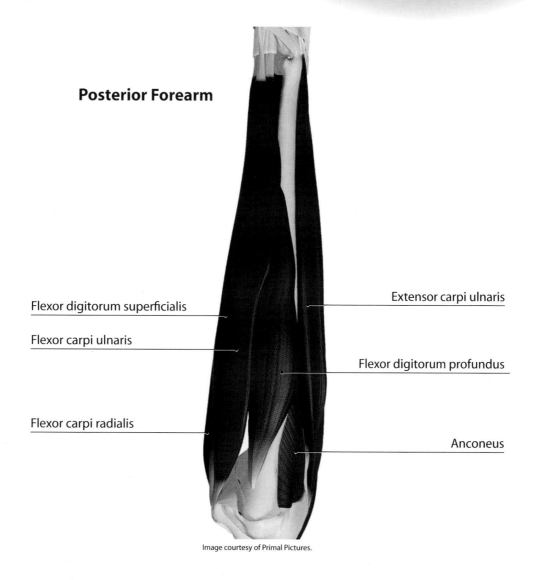

Posterior Forearm

Flexor digitorum superficialis

Flexor carpi ulnaris

Flexor carpi radialis

Extensor carpi ulnaris

Flexor digitorum profundus

Anconeus

Image courtesy of Primal Pictures.

Extensor Mechanism of the Finger

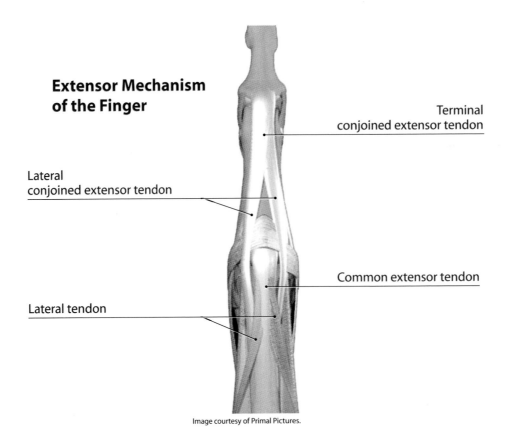

Terminal conjoined extensor tendon

Lateral conjoined extensor tendon

Common extensor tendon

Lateral tendon

Image courtesy of Primal Pictures.

Eight muscles act on the thumb to produce its remarkable dexterity. The extensor **pollicis** longus, extensor pollicis brevis, abductor pollicis longus, and flexor pollicis longus originate in the forearm. The extensor pollicis brevis and longus create a space at the base of the thumb, the **"anatomical snuffbox."** The box has clinical significance because the scaphoid bone lies within its borders; point tenderness at this site often indicates a scaphoid fracture. The flexor pollicis brevis, opponens pollicis, abductor pollicis brevis, and adductor pollicis muscles originate in the hand and create the **thenar eminence,** a soft-tissue prominence.

pollicis—Pertaining to the thumb.

anatomical snuffbox—The space at the base of the thumb created by the extensor pollicis longus and brevis tendons.

thenar eminence—Intrinsic muscles of the thumb that include the abductor pollicis brevis, flexor pollicis brevis, opponens pollicis, and the adductor pollicis.

Anatomical Snuffbox

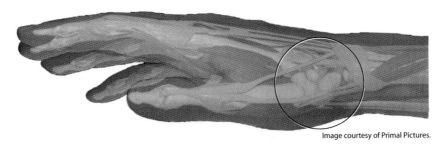

Image courtesy of Primal Pictures.

Key Palpation Landmarks

Anterior
- Pisiform bone
- Hook of hamate bone
- Thenar eminence
- Hypothenar eminence

Posterior
- Carpal bones
- Carpometacarpal joints
- Metacarpophalangeal joints
- Interphalangeal joints
- Ulnar collateral ligament of thumb

Medial
- Anatomical snuffbox
- Scaphoid bone
- Radial styloid process

Lateral
- Ulnar styloid process

Surface Anatomy

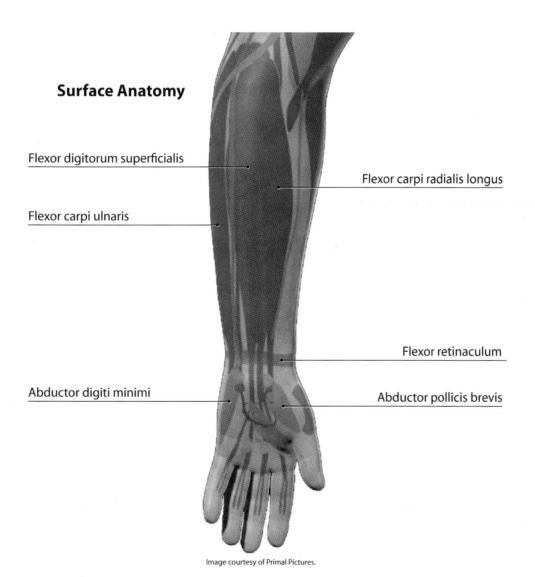

Flexor digitorum superficialis

Flexor carpi radialis longus

Flexor carpi ulnaris

Flexor retinaculum

Abductor digiti minimi

Abductor pollicis brevis

Image courtesy of Primal Pictures.

WRIST SPRAINS

Wrist sprains often occur when the athlete falls on an outstretched hand, causing the wrist either to hyperflex or to hyperextend. Be certain that you have differentiated the wrist sprain from a possible wrist fracture before allowing the athlete to return to rigorous physical activity.

Wrist Sprain Taping

Determine whether flexion, extension, or both elicit pain, and apply tape to limit the motion or motions producing discomfort. In some cases, only three or four strips of nonelastic tape around the wrist will be enough (figure 7.2). To prevent a greater range of wrist motion, however, you will have to include the hand in the procedure.

Figure 7.3 illustrates taping that limits both wrist hyperextension and hyperflexion. Place anchors around the wrist and hand and apply a base on the dorsum of the hand using three

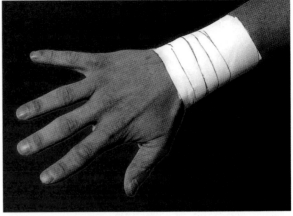

Figure 7.2   Simple wrist taping procedure to limit motion without involving the hand.

strips. Follow up by interlocking strips, in an X fashion, over the base. Repeat this procedure on the palmar aspect of the hand. You may then use either elastic or nonelastic tape, applied in a figure-eight pattern around the wrist and hand, to complete the procedure.

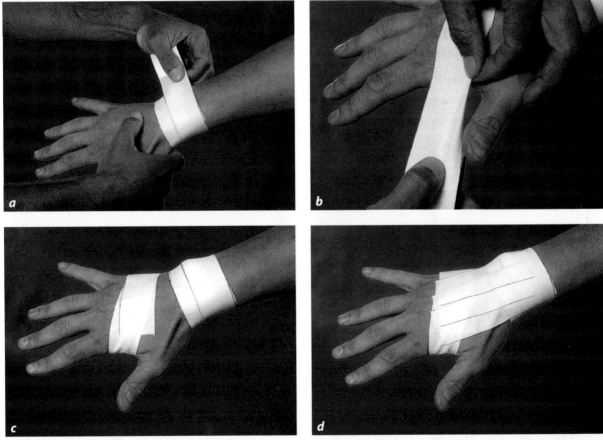

Figure 7.3   Wrist taping procedure that involves the hand to provide greater limitation of motion. *(a-c)* Begin by placing anchor strips around the wrist and hand. *(d-e)* To limit hyperflexion, place three strips and an X over the dorsum of the hand.

(continued)

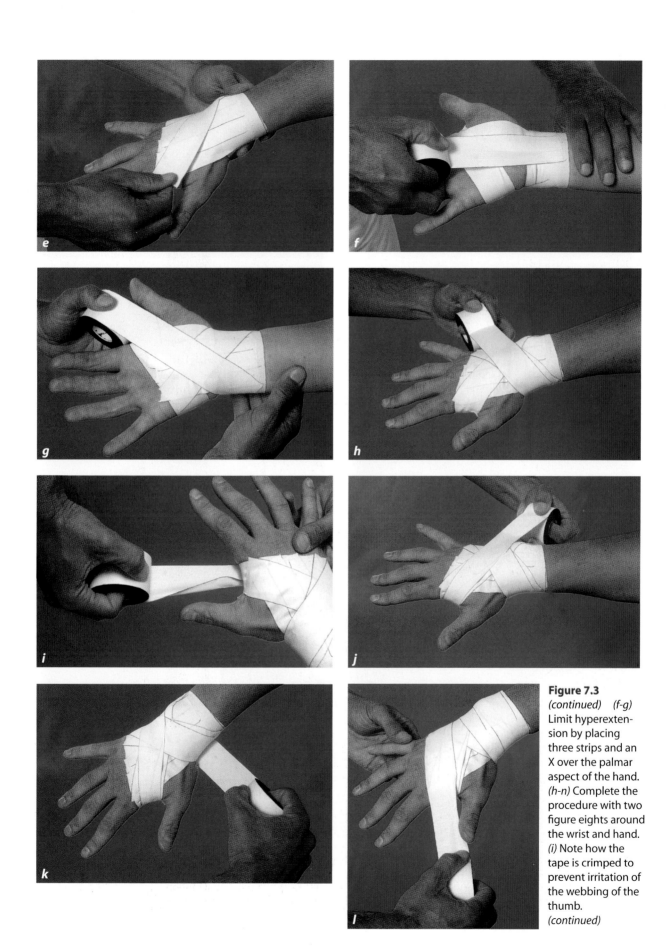

Figure 7.3
(continued) *(f-g)*
Limit hyperexten-
sion by placing
three strips and an
X over the palmar
aspect of the hand.
(h-n) Complete the
procedure with two
figure eights around
the wrist and hand.
(i) Note how the
tape is crimped to
prevent irritation of
the webbing of the
thumb.
(continued)

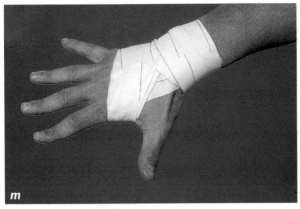

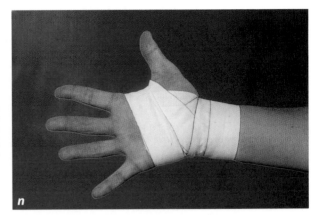

Figure 7.3 *(continued)*

Wrist Exercises

Stretch the wrist flexor and extensor muscles with assistance from the contralateral hand (figure 7.4). Hand-held weights will strengthen the flexor and extensor muscles (figure 7.5).

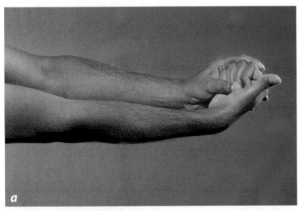

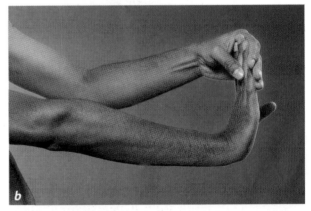

Figure 7.4   Stretching of the wrist *(a)* extensor and *(b)* flexor muscles.

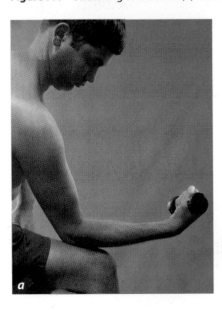

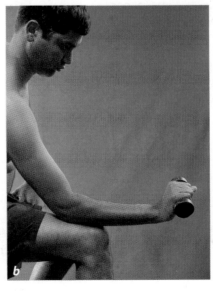

Figure 7.5   Strengthening of the wrist *(a)* flexor and *(b)* extensor muscles with a hand-held weight.

Carpal Tunnel Syndrome

People engaged in activities requiring repetitive motion of the wrist are susceptible to carpal tunnel syndrome (CTS). CTS is compression of the median nerve as it passes through the carpal tunnel of the wrist, and it causes tingling, numbness, and paresthesia in the palm, medial thumb, and first and middle fingers. Musicians, industrial and clerical workers, and even athletic trainers engaged in taping for long hours are susceptible to CTS. A brace designed to protect and rest the wrist from the repetitive stress that produces CTS is commercially available (figure 7.6).

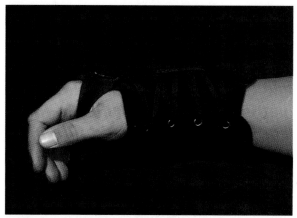

Figure 7.6 A commercially produced brace to relieve the signs and symptoms of carpal tunnel syndrome.

THUMB SPRAINS

Thumb sprains result from hyperextension and involve injury to the ulnar collateral ligament. The colloquial term for this injury is gamekeeper's thumb because the mechanism of ulnar collateral ligament injury was common in gamekeepers who attempted to break the neck of their fowl manually. Injuries that completely rupture the ulnar collateral ligament usually require surgical repair. Partial ligament tears will benefit from a taping procedure.

Thumb Sprain Taping

The athlete's pain and disability, along with the dexterity that he or she requires, will determine how you proceed. For minor injuries, a simple figure-eight taping around the thumb and wrist will suffice (figure 7.7). If the athlete needs the wrist to move freely, begin the individual strips on the anterior surface, encircle the

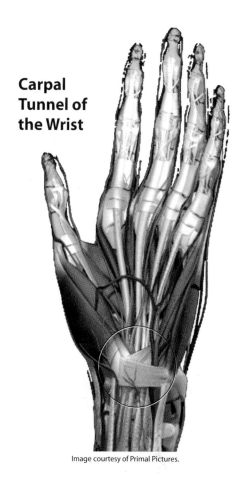

Carpal Tunnel of the Wrist

Image courtesy of Primal Pictures.

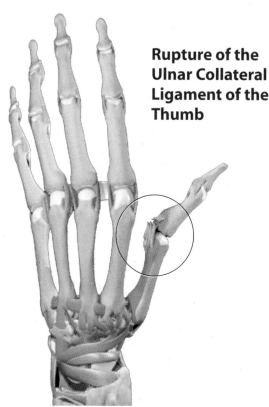

Rupture of the Ulnar Collateral Ligament of the Thumb

Image courtesy of Primal Pictures.

metacarpophalangeal joint of the thumb, and finish on the posterior aspect of the wrist.

The procedure for more significant injuries, or for athletes who do not need dexterity of the thumb, should incorporate the hand for additional support (figure 7.8). This technique requires anchors at the wrist and hand. Apply figure-eight strips around the thumb and wrist, and overlap horizontal strips from the dorsal to the palmar aspect of the hand. These strips will further stabilize the thumb against hyper-

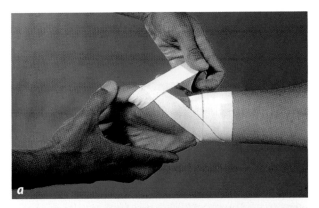

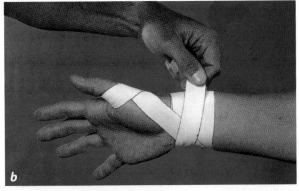

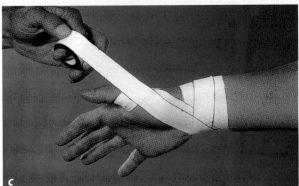

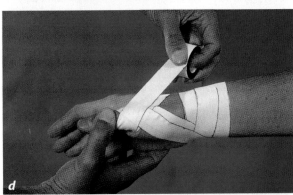

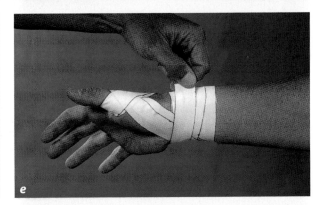

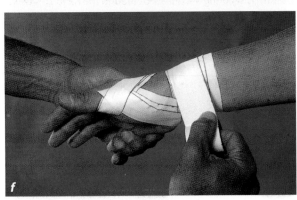

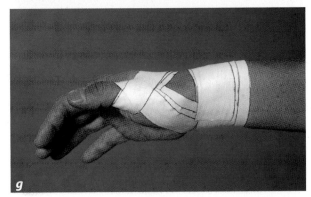

Figure 7.7   Figure-eight taping to support the metacarpophalangeal joint of the thumb. *(a)* Following application of anchor strips around the wrist, begin a strip of tape from the palmar surface of the wrist and proceed around the thumb. Adduct the thumb as the strip passes toward the dorsal surface of the wrist. *(b)* To prevent the bulk that will result from continuous strips around the wrist, individually apply the figure-eight strips. *(c-e)* Successive figure-eight strips overlap the preceding strips in a staircase fashion. *(f-g)* Anchor strips around the wrist complete the procedure.

extension. Complete the procedure with two or three additional figure-eight strips around the thumb and wrist. I do not recommend taping the thumb to the index finger because additional trauma has the potential of injuring the otherwise healthy digit.

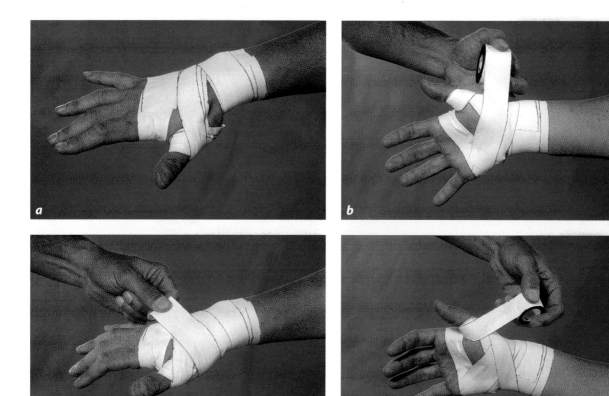

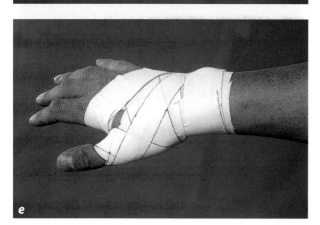

Figure 7.8 Supplement the thumb figure-eight taping procedure with tape that incorporates the hand. *(a)* Following placement of an anchor strip around the hand, *(b-c)* apply strips from the palmar to dorsal hand anchors over the metacarpophalangeal joint of the thumb. *(d)* Secure these strips with additional figure-eight strips and *(e)* complete the procedure by securing anchor strips around the hand and wrist.

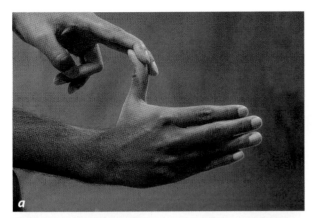

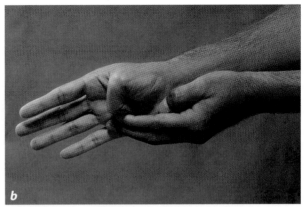

Figure 7.9 Stretching of the thumb *(a)* flexor and *(b)* extensor muscles.

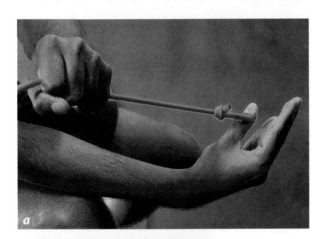

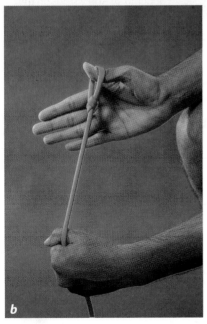

Figure 7.10
Strengthening
exercises for the
thumb *(a)* flexor
and *(b)* extensor
muscles with
elastic tubing.

Thumb Exercises

Use the contralateral hand to stretch the muscles
acting on the thumb (figure 7.9). Elastic tubing
provide an ideal form of resistance for strengthening the thumb and fingers (figure 7.10).

FINGER SPRAINS

The proximal and distal interphalangeal joints
sprain quite frequently, and their dislocation is
the most common form of dislocation injury
among athletes. Carefully evaluate finger sprains
to make certain that you do not misjudge the
injury simply as a jammed finger. Mismanaged
fractures, ligament tears, and tendon avulsions
will cause significant hand dysfunction.

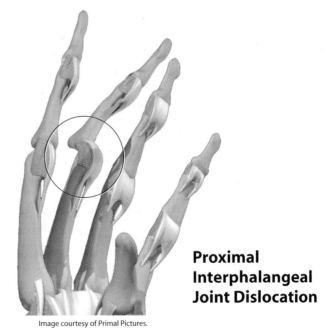

**Proximal
Interphalangeal
Joint Dislocation**

Image courtesy of Primal Pictures.

Finger Sprain Taping

Support unstable fingers by "buddy taping" them to a healthy, adjacent finger (figure 7.11). Tape around the shafts of the proximal and distal phalanges to permit movement at the DIP and PIP joints. If the athlete requires gloves, use a collateral ligament taping procedure similar to that illustrated for the knee (chapter 3). Apply proximal and distal anchors for this technique and continue with interlocking strips, in an X pattern, over the injured ligament (figure 7.12). You will need to tear 1-inch (2.5-centimeter) tape into smaller widths for this procedure.

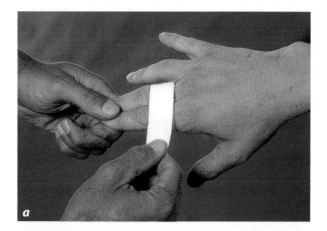

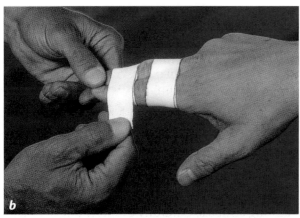

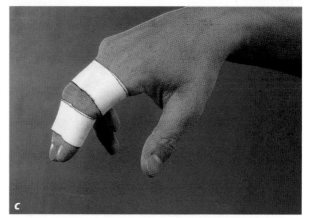

Figure 7.11 Finger "buddy taping." Support the injured finger by taping it to the adjacent finger. *(a-b)* Apply strips on the proximal and middle phalanx. *(c)* Note how the proximal interphalangeal (PIP) and distal interphalangeal (DIP) joints are left open to permit some motion of the fingers while providing support.

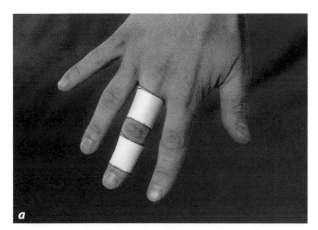

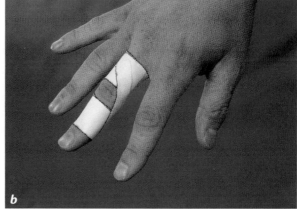

Figure 7.12 Taping for the collateral ligament of a finger. *(a)* Begin with anchor strips on the proximal and distal finger.

(continued)

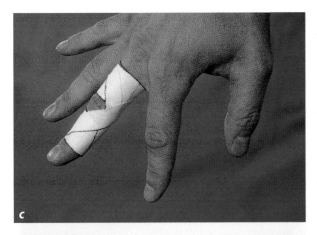

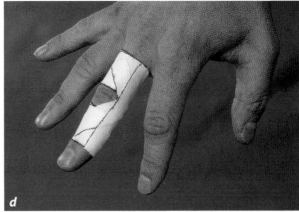

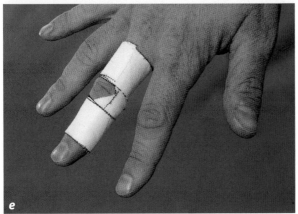

Figure 7.12   *(continued)   (b-d)* Create an X over the collateral ligament with three strips of tape. *(e)* Secure the tape with proximal and distal anchors.

Finger Exercises

Stretching and strengthening exercises employ the contralateral hand and elastic tubing, respectively (figures 7.13 and 7.14). Squeezing a tennis ball or racquetball will also strengthen the finger flexor muscles.

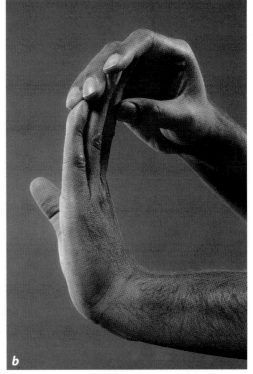

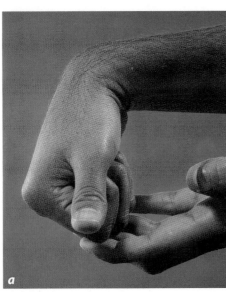

Figure 7.13   Stretching of the finger *(a)* extensor and *(b)* flexor muscles.

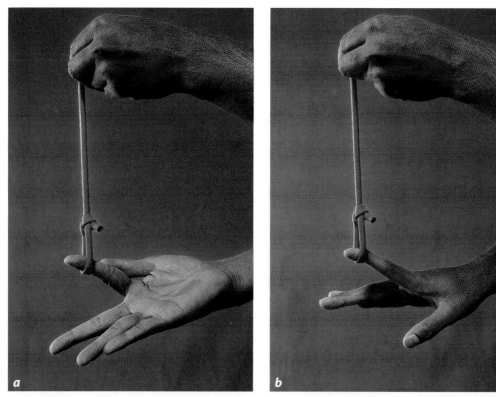

Figure 7.14   Strengthening of the finger *(a)* extensor and *(b)* flexor muscles with elastic tubing.

TENDON RUPTURES AND AVULSIONS

Avulsion of the extensor digitorum tendon from the distal phalanx will force the DIP joint to flex. This injury, colloquially termed **baseball finger**, often occurs when a ball strikes the fingertip.

baseball finger—The colloquial term for an avulsion of the extensor digitorum tendon from the distal phalanx of the finger; also known as mallet finger.

Rupture of the Extensor Digitorum Tendon

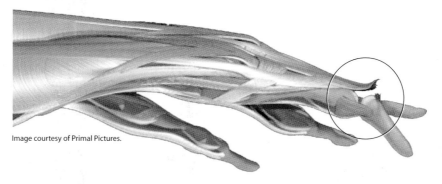

Image courtesy of Primal Pictures.

Tendon Rupture and Avulsion Splinting

Managing the rupture of the extensor digitorum tendon from the distal phalanx involves splinting the DIP in an extended position for 8 to 10 weeks (figure 7.15). Alternate the splint between the palmar and dorsal surfaces of the finger to prevent maceration of the skin. Manually extend the DIP joint while changing the splint, because any joint flexion will require you to restart the immobilization clock.

Finger Rupture and Avulsion Exercises

Have the athlete exercise the finger to restore its normal range of motion and strength after the tendon rupture or avulsion heals. Prescribe the exercises illustrated in figures 7.13 and 7.14. An experienced clinician with appropriate medical clearance should both approve the athlete to begin the exercises and provide supervision during the regimen.

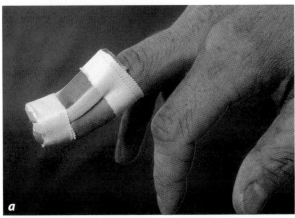

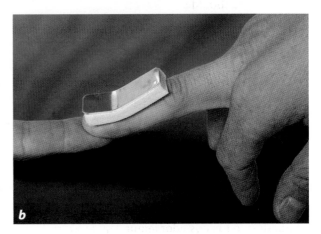

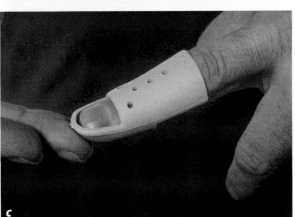

Figure 7.15 *(a)* A mallet finger splint designed to prevent flexion of the distal interphalangeal joint. *(b)* The joint must not flex while you are changing the splint. *(c)* A commercially produced splint can also be used to prevent flexion.

Glossary

abduction—Movement away from the midline of the body.

acromioclavicular joint sprain—A sprain to the acromioclavicular or coracoclavicular ligaments of the joint formed by the distal clavicle and the acromion process of the scapula; also known colloquially as a separated shoulder.

acute injury—A recent, traumatic injury.

adduction—Movement toward the midline of the body.

anatomical position—Erect position with the arms at the sides and palms of the hands facing forward.

anatomical snuffbox—The space at the base of the thumb created by the extensor pollicis longus and brevis tendons.

antalgic gait—A painful or abnormal walking or running pattern.

anterior—The front or top surface of a limb.

anterior cruciate ligament—A ligament crossing through the knee joint that attaches from the anterior tibia to the posterior femur. The anterior cruciate ligament limits anterior movement of the tibia from the femur as well as rotation of the tibia.

articulation—The point where two or more adjacent bones create a joint.

avascular—The absence of blood supply.

avulsion—The tearing away of a tendon or ligament attachment from bone.

baseball finger—The colloquial term for an avulsion of the extensor digitorum tendon from the distal phalanx of the finger; also known as mallet finger.

biofeedback—Feedback provided through visual observation or an audio tone.

bursa—A fluid sac that reduces friction between two structures.

chronic injury—A nontraumatic injury of an ongoing nature.

circumduction—A combination of abduction, adduction, flexion, and extension.

closed-chain exercise—Exercise in which the distal segment of the extremity is fixed to the ground.

contralateral—Refers to the opposite extremity.

contusion—A bruise.

dislocation—A complete separation of two articulating bones.

distal—A point on an extremity located away from the trunk.

dorsiflexion—Movement of the foot toward the upper, or dorsal, surface.

dorsum—The top of the foot or the back of the hand.

electrical muscle stimulation—Use of electrical current to induce a muscle to contract.

epicondylitis—Inflammation of an epicondyle.

eversion—Outward movement, or turning, of the foot.

exostosis—Abnormal bone growth.

extensor hood—The anatomical tendon configuration on the dorsal aspect of the finger.

extrinsic muscle—A muscle that originates in the leg or forearm and inserts into the foot or hand.

hamstrings—A muscle group in the posterior thigh consisting of the semitendinosus, semimembranosus, and biceps femoris.

hematoma—A collection of pooling blood.

human anatomy—Study of structures and the relationships among structures of the body.

iliac crest—The superior border of the iliac bone; the colloquial term for a contusion to this area is "hip pointer."

innervation—The process of sending a nerve impulse from the central nervous system to the periphery to induce a muscle to contract.

innominate bones—Two flat bones that form the pelvic girdle; each consists of an ilium, pubis, and ischium.

insertion—The point where muscle attaches to bone; usually refers to the distal attachment of the muscle.

interdigital—Located between the digits (i.e., the fingers and toes).

intrinsic muscle—A muscle that originates and inserts within the foot or hand.

inversion—Inward movement, or turning, of the foot.

lateral—Toward the outside.

mechanism of injury—Describes the specific cause of the injury.

medial—Toward the inside.

menisci—The intra-articular cartilage of the knee.

myositis ossificans—The formation of bone within a muscle that has suffered a contusion.

open-chain exercise—Exercise in which the distal segment of the extremity does not bear weight.

origin—The point where muscle attaches to bone; usually refers to the proximal attachment of the muscle.

orthotic—A commercially available insert designed to realign and alter the biomechanics of the foot.

overuse injury—Chronic injury resulting from repetitive stress.

periosteum—Outer layer of bone.

pes cavus—A foot with a high longitudinal arch.

pes planus—A foot with a flat longitudinal arch.

plantar fasciitis—Inflammation of the plantar fascia at its attachment to the calcaneus.

plantar flexion—Movement of the foot toward the bottom, or plantar, surface.

plantar neuroma—Inflammation or irritation of a plantar nerve.

pollicis—Pertaining to the thumb.

posterior—The rear or bottom surface of a limb.

pronation—Movement of the forearm to place the palm facedown; or, while non–weight bearing, a combination of dorsiflexion, eversion, and foot abduction.

proprioception—Awareness of the position of a body part in space.

proximal—A point on an extremity located near the trunk.

quadriceps (q)-angle—The degree of obliquity of the quadriceps.

quadriceps femoris—The muscle group in the anterior thigh consisting of the rectus femoris, vastus medialis, vastus intermedius, and vastus lateralis.

retinaculum—A soft-tissue fibrous structure designed to stabilize tendons or bones.

rotator cuff—The muscle group in the shoulder consisting of the subscapularis, supraspinatus, infraspinatus, and teres minor.

shin splints—A colloquial term for pain in the leg that can originate from any number of possible sources.

spica—A figure-eight wrap that incorporates the thigh and hip or the arm and shoulder.

sprain—An overstretching (first degree), partial tearing (second degree), or complete rupture (third degree) of a ligament.

static stretching—Stretching a muscle in a stationary position.

strain—An overstretching (first degree), partial tearing (second degree), or complete rupture (third degree) of any component of the muscle-tendon unit.

subluxation—A partial dislocation of a joint.

superficial—Toward the surface of the body.

supination—Movement of the forearm to place the palm faceup; or, while non–weight bearing, a combination of plantar flexion, inversion, and foot adduction.

surface anatomy—Study of the form and surface of the body.

tendinitis—Inflammation of a tendon or its sheath.

thenar eminence—Intrinsic muscles of the thumb that include the abductor pollicis brevis, flexor pollicis brevis, opponens pollicis, and the adductor pollicis.

valgus—Alignment of a joint or stress to the joint that places the distal bone in a lateral direction; the "knock-kneed" position of the knee joint.

varus—Alignment of a joint or stress to the joint that places the distal bone in a medial direction; the "bow-legged" position of the knee joint.

Suggested Readings

Denegar, C.R., S. Saliba, and E. Saliba. In press. *Therapeutic modalities for musculoskeletal injuries.* 2nd ed. Champaign, IL: Human Kinetics.

Hillman, S.K. 2005. *Introduction to athletic training.* 2nd ed. Champaign, IL: Human Kinetics.

Houglum, P.A. 2005. *Therapeutic exercise for musculoskeletal injuries.* 2nd ed. Champaign, IL: Human Kinetics.

Ray, R. 2005. *Management strategies in athletic training.* 3rd ed. Champaign, IL: Human Kinetics.

Shultz, S.J., P.A. Houglum, and D.H. Perrin. 2005. *Examination of musculoskeletal injuries.* 2nd ed. Champaign, IL: Human Kinetics.

About the Author

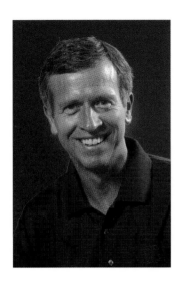

David H. Perrin, PhD, ATC, is dean and professor of the School of Health and Human Performance at the University of North Carolina at Greensboro. Before going to Greensboro, Perrin directed the athletic training program at the University of Virginia from 1986 to 2001. He received the Sayers "Bud" Miller Distinguished Educator Award from the National Athletic Trainers' Association (NATA) in 1996, the Most Distinguished Athletic Trainer Award from NATA in 1998, and was inducted into the NATA Hall of Fame in 2003. Perrin was a member of the NATA Professional Education Committee from 1982 to 1995 and was editor-in-chief of the *Journal of Athletic Training* from 1996 to 2004.

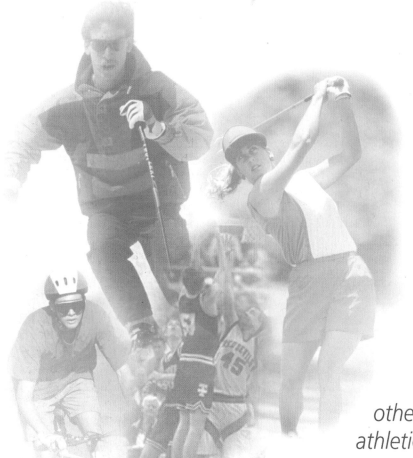